When Diabetes Complicates Your Life

Controlling Diabetes and Related Complications

Joseph Juliano, MD

CHRONIMED PUBLISHING

When Diabetes Complicates Your Life, Revised Edition: Controlling Diabetes and Related Complications
©1993, 1998 by Joseph Juliano, MD

Library of Congress Cataloging-in-Publication Data

Juliano, Joseph, MD
When diabetes complicates your life: controlling diabetes and related complications / Joseph Juliano
p.   cm.
Includes index
ISBN 978-1-62045-715-3

Edited by: Jeff Braun
Cover Design: Nancy Nies
Text Design & Production: David Enyeart
Art/Production Manager: Claire Lewis

Printed in the United States of America

Published by
Chronimed Publishing
P.O. Box 59032

Minneapolis, MN 55459-0032

10   9   8   7   6   5   4   3   2   1

Notice: Consult a Health Care Professional
Because individual cases and needs vary, readers are advised to seek the guidance of a licensed physician, registered dietitian, or other health care professional before making changes in their prescribed health care regimens. This book is intended for informational purposes only and is not for use as an alternative to appropriate medical care. While every effort has been made to ensure that the information is the most current available, new research findings, being released with increasing frequency, may invalidate some data.

This book is lovingly dedicated to my mother and father and to the person who inspired the following poem:

Glass Butterflies and Rainbows in the Dark
Dimensions in time flutter and waver
To the majestic sympathetic algorithms of reality.
But what of this time, this time of now,
This time of you, this time of me,
This dimension in time of you and me.
O brutal reality, O exquisite fantasies,
Permutations beyond glass rainbows abound,
Cry out to me not softly your dreams.
Tinsel thin glass surrounds a framework of heavy metal
As I look into her soul to witness
synchronistic chromatic colors.
Spring forth O beautiful glass butterfly.
And as you take on life blood's flow,
Emerge into the aura
And redefine the colors of rainbows in the dark for him.

Joseph Juliano

I would like to give special thanks to Charles Erickson, M.D., who gave me my first insulin injection and thus saved my life, and to William Hutton, M.D., who tried so valiantly to save my eyesight, thus giving me the will to live. Special thanks also to James S. Logan, M.D., and to Betty Taylor.

I would like to especially thank Jo Ann, Vic, Bobby, and Judy for reading the manuscript during the writing process and for adding constructive criticism, and Ed Bryant of *The Voice of the Diabetic.*

Further gratitude goes to Max Ellenberg, M.D., and Harold Rifkin, M.D., whose writings have been so important to my understanding of diabetes.

I would also like to express my thanks to my friends and family, whom I am blessed to have, for their support during the writing of this book.

CONTENTS

Preface

IT didn't take much thought to decide to write this revised edition of *When Diabetes Complicates Your Life*—especially when you consider all of the advancements in diabetes care and knowledge that have occurred since the original edition appeared in 1993.

Leading the list of breakthroughs is the Diabetes Control and Complications Trial (DCCT). This landmark study confirmed what I and many other diabetes practitioners had long believed: the devastating complications of diabetes can be prevented or delayed by keeping your blood glucose levels as normal as possible. The findings were so clear-cut that the 10-year study was halted a year early—just after the first edition of this book was published.

The book was no less relevant in light of the DCCT. The study simply provided the scientific proof and methods for maintaining tight blood glucose control. (It also exposed some problems associated with tight control, such as weight gain and a greater risk of insulin reactions, which I will discuss later in the book.) The DCCT also brought widespread attention to the impact of diabetes complications.

The past five years have produced other important advancements. New medications, improved medical equipment, and new treatment options are just a few of the topics covered in this revised edition of *When Diabetes Complicates Your Life.*

As I write this, I am in my 34th year with Type 1 diabetes. My medical education is as an endocrinologist and research scientist. My life's work has been devoted, in large part, to understanding this disease we call diabetes mellitus. This book is the culmination of 20 years of dreaming that someday I would have the time to write for the betterment of the diabetic population.

It is indeed strange that in order to have the time, I had to suffer one of the most ravaging complications of diabetes. I have been totally blind from complications of diabetic retinopathy for 14 years now.

I truly feel I have overcome this tremendous obstacle with a healthy and positive determination to make my life better and better. My goal is to share my experience in managing this disease and my success in dealing with the complications of long-term diabetes.

Throughout this book, I speak to you not only as a doctor and endocrinologist, but also as a fellow diabetic who understands only too well the ups and downs, frustrations, and suffering from living with diabetes. You will quickly note that I don't cut you much slack. Blindness, kidney disease, and other serious complications are all discussed right off the bat.

As for managing your diabetes, it's important to make healthy choices. Checking your blood glucose seems like a monumental inconvenience; however, it is not optional. In my opinion, this is one of those mandatory tasks, just like taking your insulin or taking your oral medications. I check my blood glucose two or three times each and every day, and yes, sometimes my fingertips do become tender.

I believe we diabetics really have no time for complaining about the small things. It is much more important that we understand that the finger prick will lead to better diabetic control, improved health, and less chance for complications.

It is with this attitude I would like you to read and understand this book.

You'll note I constantly stress the positive, even when I must delve into the negatives of long-term complications. Please, always keep in mind that knowledge is strength. The more you know about and understand diabetes, the more powerful your control. Your determination to strive for knowledge and understanding is a key factor to your overall health.

This book has been written as a self-help guide. Please join me in a renewed effort to treat diabetes with the ultimate in positive mind-sets. Program your mind to act as a computer that allows only the most positive thoughts to enter. We can then move toward a better understanding of this puzzling disorder called diabetes.

Joseph Juliano

When the News Hits Home

"WE received your lab results today. Your blood glucose is very high, and just as I thought, you have severe Type 1 diabetes. We will start you immediately on insulin therapy by subcutaneous injection. Depending on the protocol we choose, you will have to give yourself two to four insulin injections every day and check your blood glucose three to six times every day for the rest of your life. Now, do you have any questions?"

Perhaps this is how you were introduced to the fact you are now a diabetic. Whether you have Type 1 or Type 2 diabetes, just the thought of jabbing yourself with a needle every day for the rest of your life can make the mind reel and the stomach turn.

Not all doctors are so clinical and abrupt as in this example, but good bedside manner or not, the finality of a diagnosis of diabetes can be devastating. Along with what you may know about diabetes, plus the usual horror stories from well-meaning friends and family, the news can be frightening.

Diabetes is so prevalent, almost everyone knows someone who has the disease. Without necessarily meaning to, friends or relatives can trigger unnecessary fear. The comments often run something like this:

"Oh, my god, that is just horrible. You'll have to give yourself shots every day. Jane Smith suffered with diabetes and went blind and then lost her kidneys. Such a terrible life. The poor thing finally had an insulin reaction that killed her."

If you're newly diagnosed and have little knowledge of the disease, such horror stories can be traumatic. Certainly they don't encourage you to approach the problem positively! Yet, diabetes can be managed.

It's vitally important for every person with diabetes to understand the disease. No, this will not happen overnight. It takes time and patience. It also takes a strong desire, willingness to learn difficult tasks, and the discipline to change your lifestyle.

The term "diabetes mellitus" is of Greek derivation. Literally translated, it means "honey siphon." "Diabetes" means siphon or tube and "mellitus" means honey or sugar. Freely translated, diabetes mellitus means a running through of sugar, which certainly describes the condition well, at least in its uncontrolled state.

Throughout this book, we'll focus on Type 1 diabetes, which accounts for perhaps 10 percent of all cases in the United States. That doesn't mean people with Type 2 diabetes do not need to be concerned with complications. On the contrary, the same complications can develop as in Type 1 diabetes. Some may already be present at diagnosis. That's because the onset of Type 2 diabetes is usually much more subtle than Type 1. In fact, most people who develop Type 2 diabetes probably have had some degree of high blood glucose for years. Type 2 diabetes usually can be managed with diet and exercise. However, an estimated 40 percent of Type 2 diabetics do take insulin, and this information should be helpful for them.

I begin this book with diagnosis, because once the diagnosis is made, the healing process begins—both physically and mentally. Prompt and continuing insulin therapy is the key to a return to good health. It's a near miracle that with the very first injection of insulin, the uncontrolled diabetic begins to regain control—and regain life. Without diagnosis and treatment, an uncontrolled diabetic continues to waste away until a hyperglycemic coma sends him or her to the hospital.

In this book, our goal is to understand diabetes on a personal day-to-day basis. Together we'll work through the realities of diabetes, explore the possible long-term complications, learn about the modern tools we have available, and finally develop a healing mind-set to help us deal with the daily challenge of diabetes.

Emotions Are Important

We're all prone to daily mood swings. One morning we're so cheerful it almost makes friends cringe, yet later in the day we're capable of making others miserable. These up and down feelings are normal, as long as they don't become superhighs (manic conditions) or superlows (depression).

Moods are affected by events like losing a loved one or being laid off. But with diabetes, wide swings in blood glucose levels can also affect emotions. Varying blood glucose levels affect each of us differently.

When I run a high blood glucose level, I often become boisterous and laugh and joke. When I run a low blood glucose level, I tend to be unnaturally quiet, saying little to others. I know my personality changes with high and low blood glucose. You'll have to monitor yourself for your responses.

In some people, it's obvious by their actions whether they're experiencing high or low blood glucose. However, low blood glucose symptoms seem to be more easily recognized than high blood sugar symptoms. With low blood glucose, you may experience confusion, irritability, or emotional outbursts. Symptoms of high blood glucose are more gradual and include dry mouth, thirst, and drowsiness.

Don't ever guess your blood glucose level. I've tried guessing a week's worth of fasting morning blood glucose. How well did I predict whether I had high or low blood glucose? I was right about one in four times. And a grade of 25 percent is failing. Don't guess. The only way to determine your blood glucose level is to check it with a monitor. Even with my 30-plus years of experience with diabetes, I can't reliably guess what my blood glucose is without checking it.

No Time for Complaining

I strive to be even-tempered and good-natured. I'm not always successful, but I give myself an above-average grade. If you constantly ask people why you have diabetes and why you have to watch your diet and take insulin injections, you will be left to ponder these questions by yourself. Bitterness does indeed invite loneliness.

For now, diabetes is incurable. This realization can be difficult to grasp. Like anyone else, I get depressed and angry at times. The word "incurable" has many negative connotations. It causes fear, uncertainty, and dread of what the future might hold.

Denial is common, and it's usually what we feel at first. We deny that this disease will have any affect on us at all. But this is dangerous. We may be tempted to skip our insulin or other requirements, such as blood testing, regular visits to the doctor, and healthy eating and exercise.

Often, denial is followed by feelings of anger, guilt, or sadness. We tell ourselves it isn't fair that we've got diabetes. We don't deserve it. No one understands us.

These are all natural and understandable feelings. But we must accept diabetes and come to grips with the possibility of long-term complications.

The immediate challenge of a newly diagnosed diabetic is to learn about the disease as quickly as possible. The physician, the endocrinologist, the diabetes educator, the dietitian, family members, and the new diabetic all must work as a team to help the diabetic into a new lifestyle.

My diagnosis was missed for two years because the doctors I saw did not order blood glucose tests. Thirty-five years ago, blood chemistries and fasting-blood glucose tests were not routine. When I entered the hospital at age 15, my life changed forever. A fine young endocrinologist saw to it that the changes were for the better. He drew out some regular insulin into a syringe and gave me my first insulin injection in the abdomen. He then sat down at my bedside and patiently talked with me.

"Joe, today we have begun treatment for your diabetes. Somehow, you have turned up with this disease even though there is no diabetes in your family. We don't know how you got this disease or why. I want you to think of yourself as a doctor, because, for the rest of your life, you will have to be your own doctor. I can't possibly be with you 24 hours a day. Of course, you'll see me for visits so I can make sure you're all right. But it is up to you to control your diabetes on a daily basis.

"Diabetes is a challenge. Some fail to meet this challenge. Others manage this disease with courage and overcome the many problems that come with daily care. So, from now on, I want you to think of yourself as a special doctor with a special challenge."

I will never forget his words. The endocrinologist who so inspired me into accepting my diabetes also inspired me to go to medical school and study endocrinology and the cause of diabetes mellitus. He will never know what an important role he played in my life—unless he reads this book.

His inspiration has helped me again and again to meet the challenges of diabetes. He triggered an acceptance I have carried with me for over 30 years, even during times of extreme adversity. He handed me four books on diabetes. I read them all during my stay in the hospital. I've been studying diabetes ever since.

In this book, I call on you, the diabetic, to consider yourself a special doctor with a special challenge. I believe looking at your diabetes this way will help you carry out your doctor's directions in an especially helpful manner.

Reacting to Possible Problems

In 1985, I attended a rehabilitation school for the newly blind. Four of us who had lost our eyesight because of diabetic retinopathy decided to attend that month's meeting of the American Diabetes Association. My blind companions included an elderly gentleman, a government worker in her 30s, and a young college woman.

Using each other for emotional support, we tapped our new white canes along the hallways and found the meeting. As we came to the double-wide doorway, the group turned to see us—a widely ranging group of blind diabetics, white canes in hand, with determined looks of independence.

We waited there wondering where we would find a place to sit among the crowd. Finally, a sweet lady came to our rescue and escorted us to some chairs—in an empty row, we learned later.

The tension in the room was great. We were facing what everyone in the room probably held as their most dreaded fear—blindness. To top all of this, the lecture was on complications of diabetic retinopathy.

Fortunately, there was an opportunity for me to add my perspective to the discussion—as someone who's lived with diabetic retinopathy and been involved in the medical research of the disease. And I think we were able to relieve some of their fears by talking about how the complication arose in each one of us.

Another time, I was invited to speak to a support group for people with diabetes. They were clearly uneasy when I told them I had lost my eyesight to diabetes. I went on and spoke about the stages of retinopathy, including possible treatments.

Midway through the presentation, a woman interrupted with a question.

"Why are you telling us all of these horror stories?" she angrily asked. "I thought your talk was going to be on the positive sides of diabetes. I think you're bitter because of your handicap."

"I understand why you might feel that way," I said. "But don't shoot the messenger just because he brings news you don't want to hear.

"Retinopathy and other serious complications can occur with long-term diabetes. We don't understand all the factors, but it's important to know the realities.

"Turn your anger into positive energy. Do everything you can to manage your diabetes," I urged. "How about encouraging the government to expand diabetes research?"

The woman was not satisfied by my response and left the auditorium, followed by others.

Like that lecture, this book will tell it like it is. The first five chapters are especially hard hitting. I talk about complications that can affect your eyes, kidneys, nerves, and blood vessels. After that, however, comes information on how to best manage your diabetes and hopefully minimize or prevent complications.

You may feel like dropping this book and bolting out of the room when I discuss complications. But denying the possibility of complications won't help you; learning about them will.

Remember, knowledge is strength. The more you know about diabetes, the better your life will be.

Chapter One

My Story

BEFORE I discuss the complications of long-term diabetes, I would like you to prepare yourself mentally. What you will read is information that will set reference points for better understanding and care of this complex disease. By giving yourself the best possible daily care, it is my sincere hope and prayer that you will not have any of the long-term complications, such as kidney failure, nerve damage, and blindness.

Why does uncontrolled diabetes produce such horrible complications? For that matter, why do I have to have this disease in the first place? These are valid questions for which I have no real answers: I have asked them many times myself. With modern medical techniques, the diabetic has been afforded a longer and longer life span. By living longer, the person with diabetes now may face the complications associated with long-term diabetes.

In the early days, people with diabetes were not expected to live very long. This seems archaic, but even today, when a modern well-trained doctor diagnoses diabetes in a tribesman in a remote African village, basically all the doctor can do is send the person home to face certain eventual death from diabetic ketoacidosis, hyperglycemia, and other complications of uncontrolled diabetes. Even with insulin and syringes available, the insulin often deteriorates because of lack of refrigeration.

It is ironic that longer lives for individuals with diabetes can mean more devastating complications. This is not universal, though. Why doesn't everyone with diabetes go totally blind? Why doesn't everyone with diabetes lose kidney function and suffer leg amputations?

Medical researchers could certainly move ahead faster if all diabetics fell neatly into these categories. But diabetes does not affect everyone the same. True, diabetes is the number one cause of new blindness in the United States, but not all long-term diabetics suffer total blindness. In fact, many diabetics have only the lens stiffening caused by aging and thus require the usual remedy: reading glasses or bifocals. Some diabetics will require treatment for retinopathy (damage to the retina), but many need only basic treatment and will not lose their eyesight. Many diabetics suffer kidney failure along with diabetic eye disease, for a one-two punch that makes surviving extremely difficult. Yet I can tell you about many courageous people I know personally who have survived both of these complications.

We can search for answers to the "whys" of all this, but I have yet to find a satisfactory explanation. And let me tell you, during my initial stage with total blindness, I had many solitary moments to think about diabetes in its entirety.

I invite you to read my story—my personal account of the problems that led to total blindness. It is meant to inspire you, not to depress you.

Number One Fear

Have you ever thought about the number one health fear expressed by most Americans? It used to be cancer, followed by blindness. Now it's blindness. Cancer has slipped to the number two position.

Why do we have this fear of losing our eyesight? The answer is obvious. We depend on sight more than any other sense. The immediate question is: How would I even be able to read this book? Then there are others: I must pick up my teenager after baseball practice today, but how would I do that if I were blind? How would I balance my checkbook? How would I sort the clothes for the wash? How would I make dinner? How would I do anything if I lost my eyesight?

I asked these same questions in 1984 as my perfect 20-15 vision (better than normal 20-20) progressively deteriorated to total blindness. The experience of losing eyesight is always devastating. Our lifestyle, whatever it may be, must change. No matter what your age (after age six, when the visual cortex has developed sufficiently to create visual memory), blindness is a shocking jolt to the body's perceptual reflexes. Still, in view of my life experience, I can honestly say all is not lost. I can still do fantastic things even with total blindness.

I was diagnosed with diabetes mellitus at age 15; two doctors had missed the diagnosis two years earlier. My wise grandmother and mother noticed the fruity smell to my breath, the frequent urination, and the sticky patches around the toilet, like someone had spilled a sweet soft drink. I was building up a tremendous amount of sugar in my blood; the excess was being carried out through my urine. With five or six trips to the bathroom in the middle of the night, it is no wonder I would occasionally miss the toilet. This proved to be a blessing. Had I not begun insulin therapy immediately, I probably would have gone into a diabetic coma because of high blood glucose (hyperglycemia). I may not have survived.

I accepted the diagnosis of diabetes and became compulsive in the ritual of shot taking and, in those days, boiling the glass syringes and testing my urine. I credit the diagnosis of diabetes with leading me into the study of medicine. If I had to live with an incurable disease, then diabetes would certainly be the disease of choice, I rationalized. I was fully prepared to live with daily insulin injections, urine testing, dietary restrictions, and the healthful attitude required for successful management. Thus, I made a major lifestyle change at age 15. (Keep in mind that this was the beginning of my high school career with its social pressures, trips to the local hamburger hangout, parties, pizza, and all the changes we feel during adolescence.)

During my early high school years with diabetes, I pushed myself by getting up every morning at 4:30 to deliver the Washington Post. It was both good discipline and excellent exercise. As I became more experienced with my diabetes, I found I could do anything—from playing in the marching band to taking vigorous karate lessons.

Diabetes Education

After I graduated from college, I entered medical school. The heavy demands of reading, studying, and attending classes were very difficult at times. Sometimes I really wanted to give it up. I had to juggle meal times and shot times, often to the detriment of my diabetes. There were tests almost every day. The emotional stress, along with the physical demands, pushed me to the limits of my ability. But I made it through, somehow. I got married and moved to California to do post-graduate medical research.

I had become involved in basic clinical research into the molecular basis of diabetes while in medical school, and I continued this study in California. I gained great insight into the working diabetic's emotional state. The research was high powered and demanding, requiring more than just 40 hours a week. With the work, I attained a certain amount of financial success and became caught up in the emotional stress and pressure required to maintain a "successful" lifestyle.

In addition to careful management of my diabetes, including meticulous attention to insulin injections, exercise, and diet, I had regular checkups with an endocrinologist or an internist. My diet always included leafy vegetables and lean meats, fish, and poultry. I have never had any trouble eating more salad than the main course. I thought I was doing everything I could to control my disease.

In 1983, on a regular visit to my ophthalmologist, (a retinal specialist and friend through our mutual love of sports cars), he pronounced his finding.

"I hate like hell to tell you this," he said, swinging the slit lamp out of my way, "but you have a damn good case of retinopathy. We will have to begin laser treatments immediately—two sessions a week, beginning with the right eye, which seems to be somewhat worse than the left."

He gave me no real choice. I knew the situation only too well. But this only happened to other diabetics, not to me. I mean, why me? Hadn't I been taking care of myself?

I drove home and told my wife I would have to begin laser treatments for my diabetic retinopathy. For as long as I live, I will never forget her reaction to this bad news: "Well, if you go blind, I will divorce you." I was crushed; but I believed I would never lose my eyesight to this condition. We had found it in the nick of time, I rationalized. Modern laser therapy was well-known to save diabetics' vision. When I expressed the fear of going blind to my ophthalmologist friend, he told me how excellent my prognosis looked.

"Perhaps in seven or eight years we will have to do additional laser therapy, but we will be further along medically in understanding this condition," he said. "You have nothing to worry about. Your eyes are looking great."

Accelerating Symptoms

But, my eyes were not looking great. The intensity of the laser therapy knocked out my night vision, which had been excellent. Daily doses of vitamin A restored the night vision, but then I developed vitreous "floaters." These are actually tiny particles dislodged during the laser treatments. The particles float throughout the vitreous humor (the fluid-filled cavity in back of the lens).

One Saturday, in my eighth month of laser treatments, my wife and I went to our favorite restaurant. When the waitress brought the menus, I opened mine to look for my favorite dish. I saw only a blank page. I asked my wife if I had been given a misprinted menu. Her shocked look told me everything. The menu was printed just fine, but I couldn't see the fine print anymore. This was a gut-wrenching revelation.

How was I going to continue my work at the medical school? It demanded critical vision for distinguishing colors, writing, and tabulating data. What was I going to do if I couldn't see fine print?

On Monday morning, after I got to my office, my secretary brought me several phone messages and letters that required my signature. I studied the phone message sheet. I could make out the bold print, but I could not see my secretary's writing. Likewise, my letters appeared to be blank sheets, except for the bold medical school letterhead printed on the top. How could I admit I needed help?

I went to the nearest drug store and bought a pair of magnifying reading glasses—the first glasses I ever owned. Back at the office, I put the glasses on and tried to read the phone messages. At arm's length, I could not see the handwriting. I placed the memo sheet close up, at nose length. Just as I was beginning to read the numbers, in walked my secretary, horrified to see me with the memo sheet so close to my face. I brushed her off, saying that my eyesight had begun to change.

It had begun to change all right—change for the worse. I explained my fluctuating vision was the result of my aggressive attempt to control my blood glucose. The stress at this time was unimaginable.

Because my blood glucose was up and down, the lens of the eye, which is filled with a clear sugar solution called sorbitol, was being affected by the rise and fall of my blood glucose. It was like being on a rollercoaster ride; one day up, the next down. My vision changed in direct relationship to my emotional state.

The situation got worse. Every other day, I worked out in a neighborhood park. The park had exercise stations with a set of sit-ups, push-ups, chin-ups, leg-lifts, and the like, with

walking or jogging between stations. I was used to this training format and enjoyed it. I was now in the latter part of my
eighth month of laser treatments. On this particular morning,
about halfway through my exercise routine, I felt a fleeting
sharp pain in my right eye. When I held one hand over my
left eye, I noticed a blurred patch in the upper left part of the
right eye. I had suffered my first major vitreous hemorrhage.
This means a blood vessel in the back of the right eye was
starting to pump blood into the clear fluid between the retina,
at the back of the eye, and the lens, at the front of the eye.

I was almost panic stricken. A vitreous hemorrhage is serious and threatens eyesight if not taken care of immediately. I
called my ophthalmologist and got an appointment for the
following day. Before I went in, the left eye had also hemor-
rhaged. I couldn't see well enough to drive. I tried to drive to
my office that morning and was just barely able to get back
home without having an accident. I slid out from behind the
leather-wrapped steering wheel of my sports car, never to
drive again.

Loss of Independence

I didn't fully realize it at the time, but I wasn't only losing my
eyesight, I was losing my independence. It is truly hard to
imagine the mental anguish one undergoes when the realization hits that, for the rest of your life, you will no longer be
able to jump into your car and drive to wherever you want to
go. The next time someone asks you to run an errand or when
you just take a leisurely drive by yourself, think about how it
would be if you could no longer see to do these simple things.

My ophthalmologist told me what I already knew. Bilateral
vitreous hemorrhages were quite serious. My proliferative
retinopathy had turned into proliferative neovascularization
(the burgeoning growth of new blood vessels). Neovascularization leads directly to blindness. At this end stage of diabetic eye disease, a vitrectomy can be performed to save the
eye as a last-ditch effort. A vitrectomy is a microsurgical oper-

ation that removes the vitreous humor, along with any weak vessels, and replaces the vitreous with clear saline. The entire operation is performed through a very small opening in the eye. The operation is extremely delicate, but the success rate at the time was approximately 75 percent. I was referred to a retinal surgeon who performed vitrectomies. He evaluated me the following week. During that week, the retina in the right eye detached. I was now unable to see at all in this eye. The vitrectomy was to be performed in the left, the good eye.

Hospitalization

I entered the hospital able to see colors and make out shapes and forms. But I couldn't see well enough to make out a person's face, even at close range. The surgery took three hours. There were extensive tissue bands that grew extremely fast because of fresh blood in the vitreous. The retinal surgeon removed as much of the tissue as he could, along with the new vessels. I was having allergic reactions to the anesthesia, so he decided to finish the surgery. Two thin fibrin threads were left behind, attached to the top and bottom of the retina. After the surgery, I was violently ill. And, of course, I had no vision. The left eye, which had just been operated on, had a patch on it. The right eye was already blind.

After several days in the hospital, I was released and we were all hoping that in just a week's time, the blood would clear out of the vitreous and I would regain useful vision. My prognosis was for a return to at least 20-40 vision, good enough to read and drive.

After six weeks, I still couldn't see out of the left eye. I was weak and began experiencing extreme pain in my temple. The pain became so intense I felt as though a blood vessel had broken. I was given narcotics and told the pain was due to a glaucoma complication. The pain killers offered little relief, however. My glaucoma-affected right eye felt like a hard stone.

Tough Choices

I was offered several options. Alcohol could be injected into the optic nerve to stop the pain, cyclo-cryosurgery (a sort of freezing procedure) could be performed, or they could remove the eye. I was between a rock and a hard place. I decided to undergo the cyclo-cryotherapy.

In my situation, I was treated as an outpatient. A stainless steel probe was cooled to minus 60 degrees with liquid nitrogen. The loop end of the probe was placed in a circular pattern around my eye. The probe was left on the surface of the eye for several minutes in each location as the circle was completed. After this, my wife took me home and I writhed in pain for almost three hours. My wife was afraid I was going to die. So was I. She called my parents. It's difficult to put into words what I was feeling. However, after several days, the pressure in my right eye subsided, and the pain stopped.

As a result of the trauma to the right eye, the condition of my left eye, which we had hoped would be returning to vision, became complicated. Just as some vision was beginning to return, the two fibrin strands that had been left attached to the retina began to stretch and pull on the retina. This meant that the retina was in danger of becoming detached.

All of these complications were taking their toll. I lost 40 pounds in six weeks. I was so weak I could barely walk. I had missed so much work, my career was over. Also, during this emotionally troubling time, I discovered my group medical insurance was denying payment to the hospital to cover my surgery. The reason? The surgery was deemed unnecessary because of a pre-existing condition, namely diabetes. My medical bills, even with some of it donated by colleagues, totalled about $25,000 up to this point.

So, how do you feel when you are newly blind, out of a job, out of a career, deeply in debt with no money coming in, and living with a spouse who wants a divorce in the middle of it all? Well, if you have the strength, you pray a lot. I certainly did. You must also count on those around you to help. My wife couldn't deal with my intense suffering. I understand this now—I didn't at the time. My beloved mother and father were there to pick me up and nurture me back to health. It took time.

There were days that I could only tolerate life a minute at a time. When I had gathered up five minutes, I would go for another minute, and so on. The mental conditioning and challenge of my situation changed me forever. No, my eyesight didn't return as I had hoped, prayed, and dreamed it would. On the other hand, I'm still alive today. And I'm quite healthy, I might add.

The Message

What is the message here? While we are on this earth, if we live long enough, each of us will be presented with the ultimate challenge. It may involve the death of a loved one, the loss of a limb or a sense, or the many life events that cause us to ask God, "Why me?" But, why not me? Terrible tragedies happen to real people every hour of every day, not just to faceless people in the newspapers or on television. We really do have to take solace in our blessings. Life is fraught with challenge, and only those who can meet the challenge and overcome adversity will survive.

With rehabilitation—another story entirely—and the loving care of family and friends, I was able to meet and face the challenges of blindness. In fact, I meet them every day. I read magazines, books, and even medical journals through the use of tapes and discs. I get around with the help of a special white cane I've been trained to use, and I have a computer that allows me to gather information and to write through special artificial voice synthesis. I once believed life was over if you went blind. Now I know life can still be great! The only thing bad about being blind is you can't see.

Stories of Courage

There are so many more stories of courageous people who survive seemingly impossible challenges. One inspirational statement from a diabetic particularly made me stop and thank God for my blessings.

The words came easily. Nine years before, this gentleman, who had had diabetes for nearly 30 years, had lost his eyesight, probably in a manner similar to mine. Along with losing his eyesight, he went into renal failure and was forced into kidney dialysis three or four times a week. After several years of dialysis, a suitable transplant kidney was found, and although he suffered some setbacks because of complications, the transplanted kidney worked well. Some time later, his right leg was amputated. With diligent rehabilitation, he learned to get around with an artificial leg. Now he is facing permanent deafness because of diabetic nerve damage that is blocking nerve transmission from the ear to his brain.

This sounds pretty grim, doesn't it? It would be to this courageous diabetic, were he not cut from special cloth. His words are poignant: "I can see better with my totally blind eyes than those diabetics who are not with us today, who died early deaths since 1962, when I became diabetic. My legs walk better even though my right leg has been amputated above the knee, and my ears hear better than those who are no longer with us, even though I'm now totally deaf in one ear and have lost 50 percent of my hearing in the other."

Remember, these stories are to serve as inspiration, not to depress you. Take into account the challenges diabetics have had to deal with, and perhaps you can carry on with your life in a more positive and healthy manner.

Please don't feel I'm telling you these stories to scare you into compliance with good habits and skills. I know that doesn't work. I merely want you to be aware of the complications others have had to deal with.

Chapter Two

Nerves and Circulation

NERVE damage and general circulation problems are all-too common complications of diabetes. Fortunately, the DCCT proved that tight blood glucose control can make a difference. For the 700 or so study volunteers assigned to the intensive treatment group, the rate of nerve damage after nine years was reduced by 60 percent, compared to those who controlled blood glucose levels by standard treatment. It is also encouraging to know that the pain or discomfort associated with some forms of nerve damage often decreases with lowered and normalized blood glucose levels.

Throughout this chapter I will present specific recommendations to help you avoid or minimize nerve and circulation problems. First, though, I'd like you to think about the current status of your body and the changes that will inevitably occur. With age, our skin wrinkles, eyesight diminishes, reflexes slow, and blood vessels stiffen. All of these things begin to happen the moment we're born.

Now, introduce the diabetes factor. The total system, from stem to stern, nose to toes, will in some way be affected by the complex nature of diabetes. And, as you will learn, some systems within the body are more sensitive or more genetically predisposed to the effects of diabetes.

Peripheral Neuropathy

High blood glucose can damage nerves two ways, either directly or by constricting their flow of blood. The result can range from pain, lack of sensation, and digestive and urinary difficulties to sexual problems. This nerve damage, classified as various diabetic neuropathies, usually does not develop before 15 years of having diabetes.

Peripheral neuropathy can occur after several years of uncontrolled high blood glucose, when glucose proteins, called glycoproteins, form in the nerves, primarily those of the legs and feet. It can also strike the nerves in the hands and arms, though. When nerves are damaged, the brain can't recognize pain in that area. Imagine walking barefoot on a very hot sidewalk and not being able to feel the dangerous heat.

Nerve damage from diabetic neuropathy can lead to weakness in the muscles of the legs and feet. Because these muscles work as a system, neuropathy can lead to problems in balance and stability that may progress to other foot problems, such as hammer toes, calluses, bunions, and other foot deformities. These deformities are dangerous because of their potential for infection.

This case history illustrates some of the dangers:

While visiting her grandfather, a young girl played with miniature plastic toys around her grandfather's shoes. When called to the dinner table, the child left a tiny plastic chair inside his shoe. The grandfather had diabetes and was in poor control. He had neuropathy but tried to tough it out and not tell even his doctor.

The next morning he put his shoes on as usual and for the next several days he walked with the plastic toy in the toe of his left shoe. He didn't examine his feet every day, and the toy chair caused an injury that became infected. The infection progressed and entered the bone. Eventually, this man had to lose his leg to save his life.

As you can see, we are talking about serious possible effects here. Diabetes accounts for more than 50 percent of nonaccident-related amputations every year.

Think for one moment what it would be like to get out of bed each morning and strap on a prosthetic leg. Many diabetics will do this for the rest of their lives. How can we work to prevent such devastating problems? We need to rationally look at the ways we can prevent or reduce diabetic complications and associated problems.

Watch Your Feet

Because the feet are one of the most susceptible areas for problems caused by diabetic neuropathy, we need to give them special attention—every day.

Each day, take a close look at your feet. Examine your nailbeds and toes. Note any calluses, bunions, abrasions, nicks, or scratches. Look for signs of wear, rubbing from shoes, or areas of tenderness. Check the area above your toes for normal hair growth. Do your feet feel cold or warm? Do you have any pain when walking? Do you have signs of athlete's foot or cracking between your toes? Are your feet sensitive to hot or cold? Do you experience tingling or burning sensations in your feet? Do your ankles swell when you stand for a while?

This is the general battery of questions we must ask ourselves each and every day when we examine our feet. Incorporate this examination of your feet into your daily routine, either after bathing or showering or before you go to sleep at night. We must do this every day to become familiar with the changes we may encounter.

Most important, we want to watch for possible signs of infection such as redness or swelling. Any infection is serious. A simple blister from tight new shoes can spell disaster for the diabetic.

We also need to guard against diabetic foot ulcers, which can develop from an injury or infected area of the foot. They are crater-like depressions caused by neuropathy, poor circulation, or both. When not treated properly, such ulcers can lead to diabetic gangrene or death of the tissue. More than two million people with diabetes will develop foot ulcers during their lifetime.

In gangrene, the tissue is black, and this alone should cause immediate concern. The black tissue can be dry or wet and must be given immediate attention. Many times, amputation is necessary when gangrene is present.

When diabetes is out of control (meaning blood glucose is consistently high) the risk of infection is always present. A foot infection can begin after a minor injury because the high blood glucose impairs the white cells' ability to correct the problem. Left untreated, infections can be life-threatening.

Daily Foot Care

1. **Examine your feet carefully every day.**
2. **Clean and dry your feet every day.** Make sure the areas between your toes are cleaned and dried also.
3. **Trim the toenails carefully after taking a shower or bath.** The nails are more pliable and soft after bathing and can more easily be trimmed. If this is a difficult job for you, see a podiatrist (foot doctor) for advice.
4. **When trimming the toenails, be sure to trim straight across.** Do not trim too closely. Smooth rough edges gently with a cardboard emery board. If you are visually impaired or blind, enlist help with nail care.
5. **Apply a lubricating lotion,** such as lanolin or a lanolin-based product, to your feet. Avoid putting this lotion between your toes.
6. **Place an absorbent powder in your shoes and socks.**
7. **If your feet sweat, change both shoes and socks two or even three times a day.**
8. **Make sure your shoes fit correctly.** If your new pair is uncomfortable, take them to a shoe repair shop to have them mechanically broken in.
9. **Exercise your feet to improve circulation.**
10. **Never walk barefoot.**
11. **Avoid extremes of cold and hot.**
12. **Never use tight elastic bands or garters.**

13. **Do not use over-the-counter foot treatments,** including corn and callus removers and other remedies that use strong chemicals.
14. **See your doctor or podiatrist immediately** if you notice any unusual condition with your feet.
15. **And absolutely do not smoke.** Most amputations are in diabetics who smoke—a sad fact in light of all we now understand about smoking. More information on the dangers of smoking follows in this chapter.

Other Precautions

See your doctor at the first sign of diabetic foot ulcers or any other problem. Many doctors prescribe bed rest and foot supports, with a program of antibiotics if the ulcer appears infected. To avoid further complications, you and your doctor must keep close watch on healing.

All bruises, scratches, nicks, abrasions, cuts, swelling, or any change in the condition of your feet must be taken seriously. This doesn't mean we should panic over a scratch on the foot. But do wash the scratch with a mild antibacterial soap and apply an antibacterial ointment such as bacitracin. Then watch that this scratch heals properly and doesn't become infected.

When you visit your doctor, I suggest taking off your shoes and socks upon entering the examining room. This will remind you and the doctor to talk about your feet. Doctors sometimes forget this important area. Your doctor can easily tell if you have any neuropathy by testing for reflexes and sensation. The ankle jerk reflex with preservation of the knee jerk is the classical check for neuropathy.

A newer test utilizes a nylon monofilament that looks like a long, flexible bristle. It reveals if you have lost any feeling in your feet. A tuning fork is also used to test for vibratory sensation response. Other specialized tests are available that confirm the diagnosis of diabetic neuropathy. These tests include electromyography and nerve conduction velocity studies.

Some people might be tempted to soak their feet in warm

water, maybe even with Epsom salts, to soothe their feet or get rid of dead skin. But soaking actually dries out the skin, which then leads to cracking and peeling. That opens the door to bacteria and infections. So don't soak your feet and never hesitate to phone your doctor and explain the situation fully.

Try to catch problems early. Before putting shoes or slippers on, check them for gravel or pebbles. Look at the soles of shoes to see if a tack or staple might have gone unnoticed.

Avoiding burns: When preparing bath water, check the temperature with your hands to avoid scalding your feet. Never use hot water bottles or heating pads. I questioned this advice when I was younger, but I now realize that a hot water bottle, heating pad, even an electric blanket can cause burns when set too high and this can lead to infection. If you must use an electric blanket, set the heat control at low and turn the heat off before you go to sleep. If necessary, wear comfortable, loose socks to bed.

Treating the Pain

Neuropathy can cause a burning sensation or an acute sharp pain, often waking a diabetic at night. Treatment is difficult, although there is new hope with a drug called capsaicin, which is applied on the skin. Capsaicin is found naturally in cayenne peppers—the kind used to make Mexican salsa.

Some physicians report that vitamin B-12 injections have alleviated painful diabetic neuropathy. I know of one doctor who has had good results in elderly patients using vitamin B-12 and thiamine. Others do not believe this treatment is valid. Ask your doctor for more treatment information.

Blood Flow

In addition to nerves, we know diabetes affects blood vessels. It is among the top four risk factors for premature hardening of the arteries, or atherosclerosis and arteriosclerosis. These risk factors are diabetes, smoking, hypercholesterolemia, and hypertension.

Cigarette smoking decreases peripheral vascular blood flow (circulation in the extremities). Diabetes also decreases peripheral vascular blood flow. Combine them and you are really setting the stage for trouble.

Controlling high blood pressure or hypertension will also reduce your risk for diabetic neuropathy, kidney problems, and other complications associated with diabetes. Two-thirds of adults with diabetes have high blood pressure, or hypertension. This condition is serious because it leads to an increased risk of stroke, heart disease, and kidney and eye problems.

Hypertension rarely has any symptoms of its own, so it's important to have your blood pressure checked regularly. Acceptable blood pressure levels vary, but if it's 130/85 or higher, your health care team should help you determine the best treatment.

In addition to medication, blood pressure can be regulated through exercise and a healthy meal plan low in fat and salt.

A brilliant endocrinologist once told me: In the normal person, hardening of the arteries occurs "from the nose to the toes." In the diabetic, hardening of the arteries occurs "from the toes to the nose." Diabetics are particularly prone to this narrowing of the arteries (atherosclerosis) in the legs and feet. If you have poor circulation, you may notice a lack of hair growth on the tops of your feet, and the nails may look deformed and unhealthy.

Can poor circulation in the legs be remedied? Yes. The first step is to stop smoking. Next is exercise, followed by medication and finally, surgical bypass, if all else fails.

In cases of severe chronic wounds from peripheral vascular disease involving a large vessel, a circulatory bypass may be performed. This is to provide blood flow to an area either completely or nearly cut off from its blood supply.

If the area is "hypoxic" (lacking oxygen), the wound may

not heal. In this case high-pressure oxygen therapy may be helpful. A special hyperbaric chamber is needed for this treatment. The patient breathes 100 percent oxygen while his or her body is exposed to a hyperbaric state (barometric pressures higher than at sea level). The treatments are given daily until the wound appears to respond. When used with other treatments, including good diabetes control, hyperbaric treatments have improved the white cells' ability to fight infection. New capillary growth and tissue formation also improve.

New Healing Techniques

Researchers are studying how to manage chronic nonhealing wounds, hoping their patients can avoid amputations. This has led to an aggressive new approach to treating diabetic ulcers and other wounds that resist healing.

One of the newest treatments for diabetic ulcers is a topical gel called becaplermin that stimulates the body to grow new tissue to heal the wounds. Available by prescription, the gel is marketed under the brand name of Regranex.

At wound-healing centers across the country, diabetic foot ulcers and other nonhealing wounds from surgical procedures or trauma are treated in a logical program that is producing encouraging results. Many patients with nonhealing wounds are referred to a wound-healing clinic as a last attempt to avoid amputation. Note that 50 percent of the patients at a typical wound-healing clinic are diabetics with peripheral vascular disease.

It is estimated that 15 percent of diabetics will develop some form of chronic nonhealing wound, such as diabetic foot and leg ulcers. But with new drugs and better awareness, it is hoped that many of the 60,000 to 70,000 amputations on diabetics each year will be avoided.

Autonomic Neuropathy

Neuropathy can also affect the nerves that control internal organs, genitals, small blood vessels and sweat glands of the skin, bladder muscles, and the gastrointestinal tract. These nerves are called autonomic nerves because they control parts of your body that you do not move voluntarily.

When autonomic neuropathy strikes, a number of problems can occur such as impotence, difficulty urinating or sensing when the bladder is full, diarrhea, and stomach upset due to retention of food. Fortunately, specific forms of treatment are available for most of the disorders.

Until recently, sexual dysfunction in the diabetic was thought to be limited to men, but it has been found that women also may develop sexual dysfunction with long-term diabetes. Impotence in the diabetic man has long been recognized. It is now more fully understood.

In men, damage to the pelvic autonomic nerves can lead to a complication called retrograde ejaculation. Instead of moving forward, semen is propelled backward into the bladder. Problems of fertility and sterility must be considered if retrograde ejaculation is diagnosed in the diabetic male.

Diabetic men have a 50 to 60 percent incidence of impotence, much higher than among men in the general population. Impotence may occur any time after adolescence. If the nerves that stimulate erection are damaged, there will be no erection. Other causes of impotence include hormone imbalances, blood vessel and heart diseases, and some medications.

Men and women are at equal risk of neuropathic damage to the pelvic autonomic nerves. For women, difficulty with lubrication or difficulty reaching orgasm may be caused by decreased nerve sensitivity.

Diabetic Microangiopathy

Many books on diabetes do not include diabetic microangiopathy in their list of problems for the diabetic. However, if you understand this disease of microscopic blood vessels—microangiopathy—you will better understand diabetic kidney disease, eye disease, and other problems.

In 1936, it was discovered that vascular abnormalities existed within the delicate structures of the kidneys of diabetic patients. Later, it was found that these abnormalities were also present in other organs of the long-term diabetic. By the 1950s, a sufficient number of diabetics had survived to make studies of these abnormalities possible. Vascular specialists were beginning to understand that diabetes involves a very distinct set of complications to the blood vessels of the human body, and the term microangiopathy was coined to describe this condition.

With the development of the electron microscope, it was found that small blood vessels in long-term diabetics had a common factor—a thickening of the basement membrane found inside the blood vessel wall. Just what is a basement membrane? Basically, it is a band-like structure beneath the various skin layers. The term has been widened to include basement membranous structures of varying degrees of thickness, location, and dimensions. It was found that basement membrane thickening took place gradually over many years.

It is important to understand the progressive nature of this basement membrane thickening because it leads, ultimately, to the destructive complications found in long-term diabetes. Many facets of vascular disease and basement membrane thickening are not fully understood and research in this area is vitally important.

As we become accustomed to the daily routine of keeping diabetes under control, certain liberties and shortcuts can creep in. That certainly happened to me. Try your best not to let a lackadaisical attitude destroy your respect for diabetes. Keep in mind diabetes can sneak up on you. And remember to strive for strength through better understanding of the total diabetic condition.

Chapter Three

Kidneys

THE human kidney is an absolute marvel when you consider the fantastic job it does. The bloodstream is circulated through the two kidneys, each about the size of a clenched fist and located within the abdominal cavity. These organs form a meticulous filtration system that removes toxins and waste products from the blood.

Diabetes can damage the delicate structures of the kidneys. When they no longer function to full capacity, fluid backs up and waste products accumulate. This can lead to fluid retention called "edema," along with "toxemia," which is the build up of toxins in the blood.

Diabetic kidney disease is known as diabetic nephropathy. It was first noted that the kidneys of long-term diabetics contained abnormally thick basement membranes, which led to discovery of other abnormalities.

A process called glomerulopathy (the blockage of the tiny filters within the kidneys) is a very important part of blood vessel disease in the diabetic.

Simply put, diabetic nephropathy is the presence of protein in the urine. It is usually caused by deterioration of blood vessels. Here again the thickening of the basement membrane is the prime cause of the ultimate failure of the kidney. Diabetics are also prone to other kidney diseases, including hardening of the large arteries that supply blood to the kidneys.

It's estimated that by the time the diabetic has 15 years of life with diabetes, especially Type 1 diabetes, more than 50 percent of the kidney's tiny filters are blocked. Eventually the kidney may no longer function at all, and dialysis must be used until a donor kidney can be transplanted. Dialysis artificially removes waste products from the blood and returns "clean" blood to the person.

The good news is that you can reduce your risk of nephropathy. The DCCT showed that tight blood glucose control reduced the risk of kidney disease by 35 to 56 percent. Keeping your blood pressure under control will also help avoid the damage that hypertension can cause to the delicate filters in the kidneys.

Day-to-Day Care

To maintain the health of your kidneys, you must take an aggressive role in the management of your diabetes. Again, it is important to work hard to normalize the blood glucose as much as possible to prolong the life of the diabetic kidney. Also, a nutritious diet low in fat, sodium, and protein and high in soluble and insoluble fiber will promote a healthy vascular system and help keep blood glucose more in the normal range.

Drinking a lot of clean water will help flush your body of impurities that may interfere with the working of the diabetic kidney. Once you start drinking clean water (water filtered or purified to remove chemicals), you will enjoy drinking water. You may even think of drinking water before running for that diet soda several times a day. Good clean water is good for your health.

Maybe you have heard about the wonders of cranberry juice. It does seem to help many people avoid kidney problems. Actually, the benefits may be psychological; however, I like the taste and hope it will keep my kidneys and urinary tract clean. Watch your intake of cranberry juice, though, as it contains natural fruit sugar. The sugar-free version probably is best.

Dialysis

There are two treatment options if nephropathy advances to the point where the kidneys are failing: dialysis and kidney transplantation.

One type of dialysis is hemodialysis. With this method, a simple surgical procedure is first performed to create a "fistula" in the forearm. This provides the entryway for the dialysis tubing. This fistula is kept clean and is washed with heparin, which removes any clotted blood. Again, a team-management approach is necessary here for the best results. The internist or endocrinologist, the nephrologist or kidney specialist, the dialysis nurse, and the diabetic must all work together for the best results.

Each dialysis treatment may last up to five hours or more, depending on body weight and other factors, and may be required three or four times per week. Blood urea nitrogen (BUN) and creatinine clearance are carefully monitored to calculate how well the blood is being "cleaned." Blood glucose testing is also done to make sure the levels are not too high or too low.

Some diabetics with kidney failure still urinate, indicating there may be some remaining kidney function. This is usually not sufficient to properly rid the body of waste, but it may mean dialysis can be done less frequently.

More Freedom

Fortunately, today there are several new types of dialysis available. These are geared for the world we live in and allow a great deal of freedom. However, their success still depends on following detailed instructions.

One procedure uses a relatively new type of dialysis called continuous ambulatory peritoneal dialysis (CAPD). It is a home therapy in which the patient's peritoneal sac (a membrane that lines the abdominal cavity) is used to remove waste products and extra fluid from the body.

An indwelling catheter is surgically placed through the abdominal wall, and dialysis solution is allowed to flow into the body through the catheter. The solution remains inside the peritoneum for four to eight hours while the patient goes about his or her daily routine. Waste products and extra fluid then flow out through the catheter. Fresh dialysis solution is prepared and infused after each four- to eight-hour period. This is continued three to four times daily.

CAPD requires special training in order to carry the procedure out correctly. Meticulous cleanliness and sterile technique must be followed for this type of dialysis. There are special ultraviolet light exchange tools you must learn to use to prevent bacteria from entering the peritoneum. Should bacteria enter the peritoneal cavity, serious infection could occur because the peritoneum is a sterile cavity with no white blood cells to fight infections.

With patience and exacting attention to detail, it is possible for most diabetics, sighted or not, to be able to use this technique. Special adaptive aids are available for people with visual impairment. However, loss of sensation in the fingers can be a problem with CAPD.

One of the benefits to this type of dialysis is that insulin is given directly into the indwelling catheter, so injections might no longer be necessary. In my opinion, it is best if you have a partner trained to assist with this type of dialysis. Discuss the pros and cons of any type of dialysis with your doctor.

A newer type of peritoneal dialysis, called continuous cycling peritoneal dialysis (CCPD) is becoming more popular for some people. This type of dialysis is done at night while the patient is asleep. This frees the daytime for normal activities.

Transplantation

Dialysis has extended the lives of many people. And now, through better and better microsurgical techniques, more dialysis patients are candidates for kidney transplants. Not too long ago, diabetics were considered poor risks for transplants, but better antirejection drugs, improved surgical techniques, and better understanding of how to take care of diabetes has changed all that.

To combat other complications associated with diabetes, doctors are performing more and more pancreas transplants in conjunction with kidney transplants. The transplant recipients already need immunosuppressive drugs to protect their kidney, so the pancreas transplant causes no additional drug risks. Still, these drugs often have serious side effects.

In this complicated surgery, healthy pancreas tissue (usually from a family member) is transplanted into a person with diabetes. Once the tissue begins producing insulin, the patient becomes almost nondiabetic. I say almost because careful blood glucose checks must be done to make sure the organ is delivering insulin and maintaining normal blood glucose values. Many long-term diabetics who have suffered renal failure and are candidates for a kidney transplant choose this double surgery. This is a difficult decision, though, because the survival rate, while improving steadily, is still far from 100 percent.

Beta cell transplants remain a major research effort. These cells make insulin. But successful results are still far off. Researchers are working to isolate beta cells and prevent their rejection once transplanted. Experiments have shown some success in dogs, but a successful human test is not close at hand.

The surgery practiced today is so highly advanced that it goes far beyond a discussion here. I mention transplant surgery only as a point of interest and education.

The long-term impact of pancreas transplants in diabetics is not known. Will a new pancreas protect a diabetic from further complications? Unfortunately, it may take many years to discover the answer.

A 'Model' Diabetic

Caroline was diagnosed with Type 1 diabetes at age 6, after she lapsed into a coma caused by high blood glucose. Three days later she regained consciousness and dutifully began her life with insulin injections and, in those days, urine glucose testing. A very pretty young lady, Caroline became a model and enjoyed life as she moved through high school and into college.

At age 22, she learned she had diabetic retinopathy, which quickly led to total blindness. This part of Caroline's story is not so unique because diabetes mellitus is the number one cause of new blindness in this country. What makes her story so interesting is that total kidney failure almost immediately followed the total blindness. To stay alive, Caroline had to have dialysis three to four times a week.

It's difficult for me to imagine the pain this caused such a young person. Not only was her sight gone, but she had to be tied to a dialysis machine for up to five hours per treatment.

As the realization of what had happened set in, Caroline became more and more depressed. She ended up confined to a nursing home. No longer wanting to live, Caroline, now in a wheelchair and believing she would never walk again, would go to sleep at night hoping and praying to never wake up. Then she refused any further dialysis treatments. She had several episodes of cardiac arrest and was near death.

Just about everyone had given up hope. But one doctor would not give up on her. This doctor told Caroline about the possibility of receiving a kidney transplant. Because she was just skin and bones at this point, the doctor told her she must gain weight and regain her strength before he could perform the kidney transplant. He even made Caroline sign a contract that she would return to dialysis and work toward good health.

As Caroline fought for her life, a suitable donor kidney became available. Even though Caroline was considered high risk, the transplant surgery went well, and she still has the kidney today.

I met Caroline at a rehabilitation center for the blind and found a very courageous young lady. Although her bones are still brittle and she must take a number of antirejection drugs, high doses of calcium, and twice-daily insulin shots, Caroline is a true survivor.

I wanted to tell Caroline's story because such experiences would make most of us shrink into the woodwork. I'm inspired by her progress and willingness to work harder and harder every day to survive with diabetes. The one-two punch of blindness and kidney failure does not happen to all diabetics. But when it does happen, it certainly requires every ounce of strength imaginable to deal with it.

Chapter Four
Eyes

I F you read my story from the beginning, you know the risks diabetes presents for the eyes. Retinopathy is one of the most common eye disorders. It is a progressive disease believed to be caused, in part, by lack of oxygen in the eye. Because basement membrane thickens in the vessels that supply blood and oxygen to the eye, the oxygen transfer is diminished. The small blood vessels send out new weaker vessels to compensate. Their weight adds an additional strain on the retina, which is attached to the back of the eye.

Diabetic retinopathy represents a tremendous health risk. But please remember that although diabetes causes much of the new blindness in this country, not all diabetics will develop retinopathy or lose their eyesight. Some may have a slight loss of vision, while others may suffer total blindness. Each case of diabetes is individual and unique, so no one really knows how the disease will progress.

We do know, however, that keeping blood glucose levels close to normal reduces the risk of eye problems. In the DCCT, tight blood glucose control reduced diabetic retinopathy by 76 percent.

What does this mean for you? Well, consider again the fact that in the days before insulin, diabetic retinopathy was virtually unknown and there were few, if any, cases of diabetic blindness. With the discovery of insulin in 1921, people with diabetes began to live long enough to develop complications.

The relative risk of blindness is quite high among the diabetic population. The incidence is greatest for those 30 to 50 years old. In this age category, blindness is 28 times higher for diabetics and more than 88 times greater for those diabetics who have been diagnosed with retinopathy than the general population. Although these statistics are frightening, diabetes in and of itself does not necessarily lead to blindness. It is important for you to carefully understand the distinction here.

Diabetic retinopathy can be broken down into two separate categories. The not-so-bad type of retinopathy is called non-proliferative retinopathy. It is characterized by blocking of small blood vessels in the retina, which causes other blood vessels to widen and leak. Researchers have found that this type of nonproliferative disease in Type 1 diabetics occurs at the rate of about 10 percent after 10 years with the disease, 50 percent after the first 15 years, and 90 percent after 25 years' experience with diabetes.

The more serious type of retinopathy for persons with diabetes is the proliferative type. It causes a host of complications, such as neovascularization (the formation of new vessels) that leads almost inevitably to loss of sight. This new vessel growth arises from the optic disk and surface of the retina. These new vessels are weak and form a circular or loop configuration. As these new vessels add weight to the retina, which is already weakened, the traction can result in partial or total detachment of the retina. At this stage, the likelihood of retaining vision is certainly in question.

The stress on the vessels eventually causes them to hemorrhage, thus filling the vitreous with additional blood. (The vitreous is the clear jelly-like fluid that fills the space, called the vitreous humor, between the retina at the back of the eye and the lens located near the front of the eye.) When vitreous hemorrhage occurs, this new blood causes more complications. It becomes more difficult to see clear images through the vitreous. This condition also makes it difficult for an ophthalmologist to see the back of the eye.

Treatments

One of the most successful treatments for diabetic retinopathy is pan-retinal photocoagulation, a light therapy using an argon laser. The argon laser was introduced in 1968 and over the years has been refined for treating diabetic retinopathy. The procedure, performed by an ophthalmologist, is virtually painless; no anesthesia is required except anesthetic eye drops. The laser is focused through the dilated pupil to the retina in the back of the eye. When the laser light hits vessels on the surface of the retina, the heat causes a reaction similar to frying an egg. The heat destroys the leaky vessels, decreases retinal hemorrhages, and stops the growth of new vessels on and around the retina.

With more complicated eye diseases, a surgical procedure called vitrectomy can be performed. In this operation, a special needle device is inserted into the central vitreous of the eye. This device has a cutting needle and both infusion and suction capabilities. It is powered by a motor drive located on the handle of the instrument itself. The surgeon can remove blood and tissue, including vascular membranes and fibrous bands, and replaces them with a fresh clear saline solution. The saline solution allows clear transmission of light to the retina.

The most successful vitrectomies have been in individuals with blindness primarily from hemorrhage into the vitreous humor or when membranes and fibrous tissue prevent light from reaching the retina. If the retina is severely damaged, vitrectomy does not have a high success rate.

Future Advancements

Medical advances, especially in drug therapy, hold great promise for improving the treatment of diabetic eye disease. Better still, scientists are learning a great deal about preventing diabetic retinopathy.

The new generation of aldose reductase inhibitors and amino guanidine show promise for reducing the incidence of diabetic eye disease. These drugs have been tested for their ability to block the harmful effects of excess glucose on the blood vessels.

Interestingly, retinal specialists and eye surgeons generally agree that the state of the art for laser therapy and microsurgical vitrectomy is at hand. These techniques have been perfected through years of clinical practice. New instruments and refined lighting within the eye have greatly improved the success of eye surgery.

Reducing Risks

Beyond surgery and advanced drug therapy for long-term complications, what can we do, as individuals living with diabetes, to enrich our future?

In my opinion, we must do everything we possibly can to improve our overall health. It's important to have your eyes checked once a year, preferably by a retinal specialist. Of course, you must follow your doctor's recommendations concerning insulin, diet, and exercise. And checking blood sugar is a requirement, not just a recommendation.

I believe the newly diagnosed diabetic must learn discipline from the outset. By learning to keep blood glucose within the normal range, retinopathy may be prevented entirely, or at least minimized. This requires a great deal of attention to details. Make up your mind that you are going to do all that is humanly possible to prevent diabetic retinopathy. I'm not suggesting we become slaves to diabetes. However, as the DCCT proved, maintaining normal blood sugars greatly improves chances for preventing retinopathy.

If you already have retinopathy, I'm sure you're frightened and perhaps confused. But remember, action is your best ally. You, your endocrinologist or internist, and your ophthalmologist need to develop a detailed action plan—and then move ahead quickly when changes occur.

After the diagnosis of retinopathy, it is vital that your blood glucose is under control. If this means checking yourself into a hospital, then by all means do it. Your stress level will tend to interfere with blood glucose control, and it will require even more discipline and perhaps more insulin to get your diabetes under control.

Positive visualization and use of positive mind-sets, which I discuss in greater detail in Chapter 14, may also help you toward better health. Aristotle and Hippocrates both theorized that the mind heals the body. Perhaps this model of mind-over-matter will be more carefully evaluated by medical science for the future of our planet. You must see clearly the visual image of total health. Even if this ideal state is not achieved, you will feel better, no matter what the future holds.

Chapter Five

Lows, Highs, and Deadly Acids

A N insulin reaction, or hypoglycemic episode, means blood glucose is too low. It occurs because there is too much insulin working on the glucose available in the bloodstream. You will become very familiar with the insulin reaction because it is a common occurrence in diabetes.

An insulin reaction should not be considered abnormal in good management of diabetes. As you strive to maintain your blood glucose near normal, 70 to 110 mg/dl (3.9 to 6.1 mmol/L*), the tendency to fall below these levels gets higher. In other words, as you tightly control your diabetes, your blood glucose might fall below normal values and plunge you into an insulin reaction. For participants in the DCCT study, tight control meant a threefold higher risk of hypoglycemia.

It would be great if you didn't have to undergo insulin reactions, but the reaction is a fact of life in diabetes. Although it is common, an insulin reaction can become dangerous if it isn't recognized and treated promptly.

When I was in medical school, a distinguished professor presented the lecture series on diabetes. Every time he got to

---

*Outside the United States, blood glucose is often measured in millimols per liter (mmol/L). To convert a test result in mg/dl to mmol/L, simply divide the number by 18.

the section on insulin shock, he would pause for a few seconds, then say, "Ladies and gentlemen, boys and girls, dying time is near." He was very serious during this talk about insulin shock, coma, and death. At first I laughed when he used this statement. But later I learned his son had died from an insulin reaction.

Treating Insulin Reactions

It's vitally important to treat an insulin reaction as soon as possible. Signs of a reaction are sweating, mental confusion, dizziness, disorientation, and blurred vision. These tend to get worse the longer the reaction lasts.

If you are experiencing an insulin reaction, you need to consume something that contains glucose. But don't overdo it. The usual recommendation is to eat a food containing 10 to 15 grams of simple carbohydrate. Examples of appropriate choices include six ounces of regular soda, two tablespoons of raisins, or commercially prepared glucose tablets or gels, which are available at pharmacies.

After taking your simple glucose treatment, test your blood after 15 minutes. If you still have low blood glucose, eat another 10 to 15 grams of carbohydrate.

My best suggestion as an antidote to insulin reactions: Get yourself a case of those small boxes of real orange juice, the ones with a little straw on the side for easy sipping during an insulin reaction. To my knowledge, orange juice is the best and quickest remedy outside of direct intravenous glucose. Keep the juice anywhere you might need it; I always have two at my bedside. I keep them in the car, in my briefcase, and just about everywhere I go. And yes, I've had to stick that little straw into the box of orange juice in some very embarrassing places. I just shrug it off and give everyone the impression that I am a health food freak in need of a vitamin C fix.

If anyone ever asks (and no one ever has), I will tell them that I am entering a downward trend in my blood glucose that could lead to a complicated state of extreme hypoglycemia.

It's important to let someone know if you have an impending insulin reaction and need some assistance. Most people are only too happy to be helpful in an event as serious as this.

If the insulin reaction goes untreated, it can lead to convulsions, frothing at the mouth, and locked jaws. At this point, intravenous glucose is necessary and the emergency medical services must be called.

Glucagon is a hormone that raises blood glucose. It can be life-saving in severe insulin shock, so you should have a glucagon kit available at all times. Talk to your doctor about getting a prescription for the kit. Then teach family members how to inject the glucagon if you become unconscious.

One type of glucagon preparation comes in two vials with stoppers like those on your insulin vials. One of the vials holds dry glucagon, the other sterile water. After mixing, this combined solution is drawn into the syringe for injection into the person having an insulin reaction. Premixed glucagon syringe kits are also available now.

At the point of needing a glucagon injection, most diabetics will be unable to do this procedure. So, it's important to train a family member, spouse, girlfriend or boyfriend, or roommate on this life-saving procedure. Ask your doctor for a prescription for glucagon and instructions on how to use it.

If the reaction is severe enough to cause convulsions and the diabetic is still not treated, the next stage is hypoglycemic coma. The diabetic is facing impending death if emergency room treatment is not immediately forthcoming. In the comatose state, the body is shutting down to preserve glucose. When there is no glucose left for the brain, coma begins.

The First Reaction

When you have your first insulin reaction, try to remember and write down the feelings and symptoms. This will set reference points for insulin reactions you may have in the future. During my first serious insulin reaction, I was looking for the endocrinology department at Tripler Army Medical

Center in Hawaii. Tripler is a huge military hospital, and it was my first visit. After walking the quarter mile from the parking lot, I began walking the halls to find the endocrine clinic. My chest was getting sweaty, and the more I walked the halls, the more confused I became. Suddenly I realized I was having my first serious insulin reaction.

Other insulin reactions had occurred during high school but were not serious. Because I was living at home with my mother and father, plenty of food was always available. But at this first and most serious reaction, I was by myself in Hawaii and on a college student's budget. I considered the best way for me to understand the feelings associated with hypoglycemia was to live with the insulin reaction for a little while. I finally spotted a candy machine and ate two chocolate bars without even taking a breath. I got to the endocrine clinic just in time for my appointment.

I told my new doctor that I had just experienced my first serious insulin reaction and that I stayed in it for a while. He immediately frowned and warned me that an insulin reaction is dangerous. I guess I knew that, but I needed to know how I felt during a more serious insulin reaction. He just looked at me as though I were crazy and then he got on with the business of getting to know me and my medical history.

It has been a long time since that day in Hawaii. Please do not misunderstand what I am trying to tell you here. Certainly an insulin reaction is to be avoided. Now that I have a vast amount of experience with diabetes, I tend to agree with the endocrinologist I saw that day.

You can die from low blood glucose a lot faster than you can from high blood glucose. Needless to say, try to avoid low blood glucose and take adequate steps to prepare for the unsuspected insulin reaction. Here's how to prepare.

Emergency Preparations

Check your blood glucose regularly. Keep an adequate supply of insulin and insulin syringes with you at all times. Get proper exercise, and follow a healthy meal plan.

Most important, always keep an adequate supply of candy, sugar, orange juice, or glucose gel or tablets in your pockets or purse. You never know when an insulin reaction may occur because of stress, eating less than normal, additional exercise, or unforeseen problems such as having to park farther from your destination than you had planned.

Hyperglycemia

On the reverse side of the coin from hypoglycemia is hyperglycemia or high blood glucose. Think of hypoglycemia and hyperglycemia as a double-edged sword. Remember, with hypoglycemia you can lapse into coma when your blood glucose falls dangerously low. With prolonged hyperglycemia, coma may also be the end result. Obviously, the middle ground is where the ideal blood glucose should be, as near to normal levels as possible.

Even if you are taking your daily insulin injections, you may become hyperglycemic. You can usually reverse this by checking blood glucose and injecting additional insulin to regain control. If you continue to have high blood sugar three or more times per day for several days, call your doctor or diabetes educator. Maybe you're out of control because of stress or an infection you're unaware of; your doctor's objective thinking is needed to help solve any problems.

Diabetic Ketoacidosis

Ketoacidosis refers to an accumulation of ketonic acid in the body. Ketones are formed when the body uses fat instead of glucose for energy. Because this is an acidic condition, the fine mechanisms that keep the body in balance between acidity and alkalinity are upset. When this acidity overwhelms the checks and balances built into the body's protective mechanisms, the blood becomes acidic. This acid condition is not compatible with good health, and if it persists, it is incompatible with life.

If you have diabetic ketoacidosis (DKA), you will usually need to be hospitalized for stabilization. DKA happens after running high blood glucose levels over a relatively long period of time or from a sudden illness. The blood chemistry is seriously out of order, and this condition certainly requires attention from your health care team for proper return to good health. Don't attempt it on your own.

DKA is caused by an insufficient amount of insulin in a person with Type I diabetes. During DKA, your body produces an overabundance of glucagon, which is a major factor in this serious condition. Many times an infection acts as a triggering mechanism. The signs and symptoms include a semi-conscious state, unresponsiveness, rapid weak pulse, fever and flush, and usually dry skin in spite of fever.

The steps in the dangerous downward trend to DKA are as follows: Because the kidneys play a vital role in ridding the body of the accumulation of acid, they perform an all-out effort to shift the composition of the blood back to normal. The acidic blood's reaction with the kidneys produces ammonium, combined with ketones and sodium. The kidneys then excrete these acidic waste byproducts into the urine. Because the body's blood chemistry is now in a state of distress, other specialized cells are called into play. These cells produce buffers to alkalinize the acidic blood. This can lead to depletion of the cells' vital potassium.

With this flow of potassium into the bloodstream, the delicate balance is further upset, and other organs, including the heart, are affected. The kidneys respond by excreting excess potassium into the urine but this causes additional problems. If this situation continues, potassium is depleted but blood glucose continues to rise—again, as a result of chronic lack of insulin. At this point, glucose cannot enter the cells of the body, even though the liver is still pumping glucose into the blood.

With no insulin to allow glucose to enter cells, all that extra glucose is excreted in urine. If you have ever wondered why uncontrolled diabetics urinate frequently and in large quantities, this is why. Because the body is excreting large amounts of water in the form of urine, the diabetic is constantly thirsty. The loss of fluid eventually leads to dehydration.

With dehydration comes dry skin—so dry that skin tone is lost. You can pinch the skin and the resulting fold will not return to normal when released. The mucous membranes are dry, and the eyes may appear sunken. Fever is constant, even without any infection. Vomiting and nausea, partly caused by the accumulation of acid, further aggravate the situation.

Because water is vital to human life and a major component of blood, severe dehydration reduces blood volume. As the blood volume is lowered, the concentrated blood contains more and more impurities. Also, as less blood enters the kidneys, these overworked organs are further incapacitated. As you can see, the body is now toxic with its own waste, and a major effort must be made by skilled health team workers if the patient is to survive.

Treatment focuses on replacing what the body has lost. Rapid fluid replacement is begun and additional insulin, usually much more than the diabetic would typically take, is injected. A large amount of essential chemicals, trace elements, and minerals, along with drugs that alkalinize the acidic condition of the body, are given intravenously.

Any change in your health, especially infections, should be of great concern. Watch yourself carefully when you become ill. Check your blood glucose regularly. If two or more tests are over 240 mg/dl (13.3 mmol/L), test urine for ketones. Make sure the ketone chemical strips are not outdated; if the ketone test is positive, your blood is acidic. Inform your doctor immediately if your blood glucose remains high.

Chapter Six

Monitoring

YOU may not want to hear this, but in my opinion, self blood glucose monitoring is not an option. It's something you must do, along with never missing your insulin injection. It's that important for the diabetic.

"But taking my insulin injection saves my life," you may say. "Self blood glucose monitoring doesn't; it can't be as important." If this is what you're thinking, here's a lesson from my school of hard knocks.

Do you have a Commission for the Blind in your community or state? How about a kidney dialysis clinic? If you don't know and feel no need to because, after all, you are in good shape and you believe your diabetes is under control, hold it right there. If you are not aware of the local dialysis clinic or state agency for the blind, maybe you should be. If you are not monitoring your blood glucose every day, you probably will need these services in your lifetime. I apologize for being harsh, but there simply are no excuses for not monitoring your blood glucose. I make a very convincing case for this using myself as example. But first, look at a few familiar excuses:

Excuse 1: I'm simply not going to test my blood glucose. I don't want another hole in my body.

Excuse 2: No way. That lancet is painful.

Excuse 3: Why should I monitor my blood glucose? What in the world would this tell me anyway?

Excuse 4: No. I control my diabetes strictly with insulin and exercise.

Excuse 5: I just don't have time for it. It's too much of a hassle.

I used all these excuses. I'm still very healthy and quite alive. I'm in excellent shape, actually. And my diabetes is under excellent control now because I test my blood glucose two or three times every day. I'm also totally blind from complications of diabetic retinopathy. Could I have saved my eyesight by checking my blood glucose earlier? Because the nature of diabetes is not fully understood, no one can answer this question with an unequivocal 'yes' or 'no.' But for now, we have an important management tool, blood glucose monitoring, if we only use it.

Sadly, a Gallup survey in 1994 revealed that only 56 percent of diabetics monitor their blood glucose; and of those, an average of just 1.2 times per day. This is well below the American Diabetes Association guidelines which recommend that Type 1 diabetics test their blood glucose three to four times a day. Type 2 diabetics should monitor their blood glucose level one to two times a day, the ADA says.

Diabetes is best managed with insulin (or oral medications), diet, and exercise. However, without blood glucose monitoring, there's no way to know how much insulin, food, or exercise you need to keep your blood glucose in control. Serious complications may occur that can lead to death. Later in this chapter I will also discuss the hemoglobin A1c test, which can help you manage your diabetes and overall health.

Unfortunately, I can't unconditionally say you will have absolutely no problems with your diabetes if you monitor your blood glucose faithfully. But I know for a fact you have a much better chance at close control of your diabetes, thus reducing the chance of complications, by diligently monitoring blood glucose and doing everything possible to keep values near normal.

Blood glucose monitoring was one of the key aspects of the DCCT study. For nine years, people in the intensively treated group tested their blood four to seven times a day and adjusted their insulin, food intake, or activities accordingly. They even performed spot-checks once a week at 3 a.m. On the other hand, those in the conventionally treated group tested their blood once a day, but the results were not used to adjust their insulin doses. As you read earlier, the intensively treated group, which strived for normal blood glucose levels, experienced a reduction of long-term complications by up to 60 percent.

Now, frequent blood glucose monitoring is not the sole answer to reducing or minimizing complications, but it is vital to controlling diabetes. In fact, the advent of self blood glucose monitoring is the greatest advance in diabetes care since the introduction of insulin almost 80 years ago.

Strict control of diabetes is achieved through self blood glucose monitoring, careful insulin management, and a healthy meal plan and exercise program. I admit it's easy to fudge on the diabetic meal plan. Eating out, fast food, and social events sometimes make the diet hard to manage. With exercise, too often we get "gung ho" about a program for a couple of weeks or months, then let it fall by the wayside. After work, we are sometimes just too exhausted for exercise.

But, when it comes to insulin injection and blood glucose test time, there can be no fudging. You must always make time. I am talking honestly and realistically here. As a diabetic myself, I realize life is full of complexities, time schedules, deadlines, and a million other activities. However, testing your blood glucose must be as important as taking your insulin. It must be a habit—as normal as eating and sleeping.

Old and New Techniques

When I was first diagnosed, the only method we had to estimate glucose in blood was to measure the glucose in urine. This involved combining ten drops of water and five drops of urine in a test tube and adding a special tablet that changed color according to how much glucose was in the solution. We matched the color to a chart to determine the amount of glucose in the urine, from negative to plus four. Negative meant no glucose was present. Plus four was a dreaded reading we got after eating three chocolate chip cookies an hour before the test.

The trouble with the urine test is that the glucose in the urine is not necessarily a good representation of the true amount of glucose in the blood. As glucose is "spilled" out of the blood and into the urine, the percentage of blood glucose may be rising or falling, despite what the urine test indicates. If you have taken a dose of insulin, your actual blood glucose may be falling while your test results show a high percentage of glucose.

Theoretically, if you took additional insulin based on a urine glucose test, while your blood glucose was actually falling, the extra insulin could plunge you into a dangerous hypoglycemic episode—an insulin reaction. I never did like testing my urine for glucose. It always seemed like an antiquated procedure. And I was shocked at times to feel an impending insulin reaction coming on while my urine glucose showed a three or four-plus reading.

Today, by testing the fingertip capillary blood, we get a very good "relative" indication of our blood glucose level. I say relative because, first, we are sampling capillary blood from the tiny vessels some distance away from the heart and major organs and second, the instruments for home use, although very sophisticated, are not laboratory quality. (For a fasting blood glucose test, blood taken from a vein in your arm is processed by the blood chemistry laboratory. This test is a very reliable representation of your circulating blood glucose.)

Nonetheless, self blood glucose testing on capillary blood from the fingertip is the best way, at the present time, to tell where we are with blood sugar levels. Consistent blood glucose monitoring may show trends that can help the doctor or you adjust insulin doses.

Monitoring and Sick Days

Blood glucose monitoring becomes even more important when you are sick. Illness and other physical stressors such as injury, burns, and infections, cause blood glucose to increase drastically, insulin to be less effective, and, if the condition persists, toxic ketones to build up in the bloodstream.

When you are ill—especially when you are vomiting, have diarrhea, or are feverish—you should test your urine for ketones and test your blood glucose. Your doctor can help you establish a plan for handling common illnesses such as colds or the flu. It will be important to determine the amount of insulin needed, a monitoring schedule, and what foods and fluids to take during your illness.

The Finger Prick

The lancing device you use to prick your finger is razor sharp and creates a tiny hole that allows you to apply a single drop of blood to the reagent strip. This very small hole smarts a little at times. Is it a major deal? No, I don't think so. It's just a minor irritation, and with time, proper technique, and patience, we can easily get used to it—especially with today's lancing devices which are far less painful than their predecessors.

These days, there are dozens of different lancets and lancing devices. Many provide different degrees of penetration (shallow pokes hurt less) and your choice of lancet gauge width. There are even lancing devices for children.

I had been diabetic for many years before self blood glucose monitoring came into the picture. When I began testing my blood glucose, it was harder than the first time I gave myself an insulin injection. In fact, it was much harder for me to use the lancet and obtain a tiny drop of blood than anything I could remember at the time. I carefully analyzed my situation with a fellow diabetic who was a pharmacist.

I can remember his words very well. He had lost his older brother to diabetes with complications of blindness and kidney disease. The pharmacist's uncle, a former Green Beret in Vietnam, was also diabetic, and he complained that the prick of the fingertip to obtain a blood sample was just too painful. The pharmacist, who was almost fanatical in the maintenance of his diabetes, said to his uncle, "Baloney! How can a little finger prick, felt for only a few seconds, bother a tough Green Beret like you?"

This is indeed a strange psychology. Certainly the uncle underwent extreme hardship during the Vietnam experience, but he was still put off by the finger stick. So, if you feel a little intimidated by the lancing device and a drop of blood, don't let it bother you. Many others have felt exactly the same way. The tremendous benefits you will derive from better control of your diabetes far outweigh the minor inconvenience.

Monitoring Advantage

Checking your blood glucose level can affect the timing of your insulin shots. I try to take my insulin (Regular) about 30 minutes before a meal, but this is only a guideline, not gospel. Learn to be flexible with your diabetes while still remaining within the guidelines as much as possible. I realize there's a learning curve involved. You must first learn the rules concerning diabetes, guidelines, and recommendations, then learn how to live within all these parameters on a daily basis. And, yes, this can be difficult.

Let me illustrate my point with a real-life example. A friend who had diabetes recently died after going into insulin shock and coma. To this diabetic, the 30-minute guideline was a rule not to be broken under any circumstances. He took his insulin injection without checking his blood glucose and then waited 30 minutes before eating. When I protested that he must check his blood glucose, he just shrugged his shoulders and ignored me.

I tried using logic and my experience with diabetes to persuade him to check his blood glucose. Then I resorted to the rigid role of the endocrinologist, my last big weapon. Nothing would convince him that a blood glucose test before taking his insulin could tell him if he were dangerously low and that taking his insulin and waiting 30 minutes could prove disastrous. Unfortunately, he could not break himself of this habit, and he lapsed into an insulin reaction after taking his injection without checking his blood glucose. He was found two days later. He had apparently laid down to rest, feeling the insulin reaction coming on, and he never awoke. I was very angry over this, and I still am. This is a needless loss of a young person, and I hope you can learn from my experiences and the experiences of others. Monitoring your blood glucose is imperative.

Hemoglobin A1c Test

As important as self blood glucose monitoring is, clinical blood tests can provide a world of information to guide your diabetes management program. One of the most important clinical tests is a hemoglobin A1c test, which gives an average of your blood glucose levels over a three- to four-month period. It shows how much glucose has become attached to hemoglobin, a part of the red blood cells that carries oxygen.

Test methods vary among labs, so different values may be used to evaluate your test. In general, though, a good target for someone with diabetes is less than 1 percentage point above the lab's upper limit of normal. For example, if the upper limit of normal in the lab is 6 percent, the target would be less than 7 percent. In the DCCT study, there was evidence that A1c levels of 8.1 percent or lower further reduced the risk of complications.

Although hemoglobin A1c readings are not simple averages of your blood glucose levels over the past three to four months, their percentages do equate to average blood glucose levels. For instance, an A1c level of 6% means an average blood glucose level of 120 mg/dl (6.7 mmol/L); 8% is 180 mg/dl (10 mmol/L).

The Health and Public Policy Committee of the American College of Physicians recommends that the hemoglobin A1c test be performed four times per year for Type 1 diabetics, and two times per year for those with Type 2 diabetes. Exceptions to this general guideline include those who are striving for tight control using multiple injections or an insulin pump, or those who have undergone a major change in diabetes therapy.

Recently, a new test was approved for home use that measures glycated protein (fructosamine) for the previous two-week period as well as blood glucose. The manufacturer of the Duet Glucose Control Monitoring System, says it can show trends in glucose control earlier than a hemoglobin A1c test, indicating how well a diabetes management plan is working.

In addition to regularly scheduled hemoglobin A1c tests, your doctor may order a number of clinical tests ranging from cholesterol and triglyceride checks to tests that assess kidney function. Check with your doctor or diabetes team about which tests are best for you.

Regular testing accomplishes two very important things. First, it provides you and your doctor with vital information on the real status of your diabetes and your health in general. Second, it prompts you to see your doctor regularly.

Chapter Seven

Machines for Measuring Glucose

I N recent years, some of the most significant improvements in diabetes management tools have been in blood glucose monitors (or meters). New technology has made them easier to use and less costly than early models of the late 1960s.

At this time, there are over 20 blood glucose monitors for home use. Because this is an overview and not a commercial endorsement of any particular product, I won't go into detail on all the devices. I suggest you consult your doctor, nurse, diabetes educator, pharmacist, or diabetes specialty store for advice on the monitor patients and customers prefer. Your education can lead you to the best monitor for you.

Almost all monitors use light to read a chemical strip on which a drop of blood has been applied. The strip is placed in front of a light beam in the meter. The beam measures the color change produced by the glucose and displays the number on the monitor's screen. Other monitors use electrochemistry to measure the amount of energy produced when the glucose in the blood mixes with the strip's chemicals.

Some strips also change color when they react with glucose. You can match the color on a chart on the bottle of strips to get a general range of glucose levels. However, the digital reading on the monitor is more accurate than visual matching.

Monitor Operation

Most of today's glucose monitors work in the same way. You turn the monitor on and calibrate it, if needed. This is done by entering into the monitor a program number assigned to the reagent strips. You prick your finger to obtain a drop of blood and start the monitor timing while placing the blood on the reagent strip. Timing is automatic with some monitors. Depending on the monitor, it takes between 12 seconds and two minutes for the blood to react on the strip.

For some monitors, you'll need to wipe any excess blood from the strip with blotting paper when the time is up. With monitors using non-wipe technology, this step is not necessary. The strip is then placed in the meter where the light reacts to the amount of glucose on the strip and triggers a digital readout. There's nothing to it.

Some monitors store the results of 100 or more tests, including time, date, and insulin type and dosage information. Others allow their date to be downloaded into your or your health care team's computer. Even so, it's a good idea to keep a log to show your doctor at your next visit.

Many blood glucose monitors require periodic cleaning. Be sure to keep this in mind after you have used your monitor for several months. If the meter is not cleaned periodically, the reading could be inaccurate.

Check the manufacturer's guidelines for directions on cleaning your monitor. Meticulous care and cleaning of instruments ensures maximum life and dependability.

To protect my monitors, I had a special case made. A scrap of suede was custom fit to the size of my monitors, so I can take them in my medical bag or in my overnight bag without fear of damage. You can also purchase cases with the monitor.

Careful Record Keeping

Now, here's a true story. A group of people with diabetes were asked to test their blood glucose for one month, once in the morning and once in the evening, and to write down the results in a special notebook. After the 30-day period, the results were tabulated.

This research project was not intended to see how closely the diabetics kept their blood glucose in control, but it was done to check something else—their honesty.

The individuals had unknowingly been using monitors that kept their blood glucose readings in a special memory. When the actual readings stored in the memory were compared with the written results, what do you think the researchers found? That's right. The diabetics fibbed on reporting their actual test results. The researchers were surprised to find this was true with almost every person in the research project.

I could have told them this would happen. As a young person, I hated more than anything to report a high urine glucose level. Instead, I would make up a convenient negative glucose amount. I suppose this is only human nature, but it is only to your advantage to be honest about blood glucose levels.

When I first lost my eyesight, there were no blood glucose monitors that came from the factory with speech output. How does a blind diabetic test blood glucose independently? For me, at least initially, I couldn't do it by myself. I relied on help from my family. The monitor I used in those days was one I purchased when I was sighted, and I could no longer see the digital reading. Now I have a monitor that can transform the signal from the digital display to an electronic voice. This is wonderful technology!

Some blind diabetics might like to have Braille program numbers on the label of each bottle of reagent strips so they can enter this number without sighted help. Perhaps this is something manufacturers will consider for the future. This may seem like a minor issue, but many visually impaired or blind diabetics are fiercely independent and want to do as much for themselves as possible.

What Lies Ahead?

How would you like to test your blood glucose at home as often as you wish without having to stick yourself and draw blood? This noninvasive technology is being tested but it is not perfected as I write this. One example is a machine that will measure your blood glucose when you place your index finger in a hole in the machine. The small unit uses infrared light that passes through the skin to read the glucose level.

Clinical research is still being done to gain Food and Drug Administration (FDA) approval. I hope to be among the first to use it, provided it has a voice synthesis module.

Several companies and researchers are developing other types of noninvasive or minimally invasive blood glucose monitors. One is worn like a wrist watch and uses a tiny electrical current to draw body fluid into a disposable pad in the watch. It then makes the necessary calculations. Another samples the glucose level in the fluid between the cells of the body (the interstitial fluid). Work is also proceeding on an implantable glucose sensor.

A special note of caution: Please don't postpone your monitoring program because you've heard a new monitor is in the works. Delays are inevitable with any new product. And recalls aren't unusual. I suggest buying the best monitor you can afford now and using it at least twice a day. When a new technology comes along, you'll have a good back-up system.

The best diabetes management program always includes good communication with your doctor and diabetes team. It is especially important with today's high-tech medicine to use the team-management approach. But you have a responsibility to evaluate advice, practice good diabetes techniques, and become better educated in this tremendously complex subject.

Chapter Eight

Insulin Insights

DIABETES is an ancient disease mentioned in Egyptian writings believed to date back to 1550 B.C. Over the centuries, symptoms of diabetes were frequently mentioned in writings. Polyuria (frequent urination), "honey" present in the urine, thirst, fatigue, and skin eruptions have been found in early documents from India, China, Arabia, and later, Greece.

During the 16th and 17th centuries, the sweetness of urine was recognized as caused by sugar. In the late 19th and early 20th centuries, diabetes was determined to be associated with the pancreas, the endocrine system, and special cells in the pancreas (the islets of Langerhans), which secrete hormones directly into the bloodstream. A giant step forward came in 1921 when two Canadian physicians, Frederick G. Banting and Charles H. Best, discovered insulin. They were awarded the Nobel Prize for this achievement.

What Is Insulin?

Insulin is a complex, large-protein molecule produced by specialized "beta" cells in the islets of Langerhans in the pancreas. The pancreas, of course, serves many purposes in addition to secreting insulin. It's a complex organ and plays a crucial role in secretion of digestive enzymes used in the breakdown of food.

The following information briefly explains the importance of insulin. This is only a basic guide. If it sparks your interest, you may want to do more reading. The reading list at the back of this book lists resources. (I recommend Ellenberg and Rifkin in particular.)

Insulin is manufactured, stored, and secreted directly into the bloodstream by the beta cells in the pancreas. Insulin plays a vital role in breaking food down into the various components needed to produce energy and sustain life.

This complex metabolic process allows our bodies to continually make and repair cells and tissues, even when we haven't eaten for a while. Insulin is a key component needed to move glucose into the body's cells for energy and to control how much glucose is in the blood.

Specifically, insulin inhibits a process called glycogenolysis (the breakdown of animal starch) and gluconeogenesis (the formation of new glucose from protein). In this way the blood glucose is lowered through an alternate pathway.

Understanding insulin and its actions within the human body is crucial to understanding diabetes.

Types of Insulin

There are three basic categories of insulin: short-acting, intermediate-acting, and long-acting. Each is distinguished by its onset of action, peak, and duration. Onset means the time it takes the insulin to begin exerting its effect. Peak is the time insulin is working its hardest to lower blood glucose. And duration refers to how long it lasts.

The most recent development in this area is a new form of short-acting insulin: lispro. This insulin analog (a close molecular cousin to insulin) is sold under the brand name of Humalog. It starts working within minutes, permitting diabetics to eat right after injection.

The following action times are general guidelines only.

Action times vary greatly from person to person, and between animal insulin and human insulin.

Short-acting insulin, either lispro or Regular. Lispro has its onset within 5 minutes and peaks in one hour. Its usual duration is two to four hours. Regular has its onset within 30 to 60 minutes and peaks in two to four hours. Its duration is four to six hours. This insulin is clear and requires no rolling action to ensure proper mixing within the vial. Regular insulin traditionally has been used in conjunction with other insulin types. Today, it is popular to use regular insulin alone in four to six injections spread over a 24-hour period.

Generally, proper injection time of Regular insulin is 30 to 60 minutes before meals. With lispro, you can start eating almost immediately. (The manufacturer recommends eating within 15 minutes after injection.) This allows an onset interval before the insulin acts. Onset will then coincide with the ingestion of your meal, making the action of the insulin as close to normal as possible.

Intermediate-acting insulin, known as NPH or Lente, begins to work in 60 to 90 minutes. Peak action is at 8 to 12 hours, with duration of up to 24 hours. This insulin type is cloudy, and the vial must be carefully rolled in the palms of the hands to ensure good mixing. Never shake this type of insulin to mix it. Insulin is a delicate protein and should never be vigorously agitated. Shaking also produces frothing or bubbles that make it more difficult to withdraw.

Long-acting insulin, known as Ultralente, has its onset at 6 to 10 hours, peaks in 12 to 18 hours, and has a duration of 20 to 30 or more hours. Ultralente supplies a basal level of insulin and must be used with multiple doses of regular insulin. This insulin also is cloudy, and the vial should always be carefully rolled in the palms of the hands to ensure proper mixing.

A single vial preparation of premixed insulin, made up of regular insulin and NPH intermediate-acting insulin, is typically available in a 70:30 ratio—70 parts of NPH intermediate to 30 parts of regular short-acting insulin. If you were to take 30 units of this insulin, using the 70:30 ratio, you would be taking 9 units of regular insulin with 21 units of NPH. Premixed insulin is also now available in a 50:50 ratio.

I recommend carefully weighing the convenience of the single vial approach against the versatility of mixing regular and NPH insulin in separate vials. The premixed preparation is difficult for the beginner and sometimes even for the veteran diabetic to work with. By all means, check with your doctor and be sure you understand this insulin well before you and your doctor agree to use it. The premixed insulin is cloudy because it contains NPH. The same care is needed as with other cloudy-appearing insulins.

Remember, regular insulin is always clear. If it appears slightly cloudy, don't use it. How does a blind person know which insulin is which? Take a close look at the shapes of the various vials of insulin. They are shaped differently to help you make sure you're taking the right amount and the right type of insulin.

Insulin Improvements

Over many years, techniques for purifying insulin have vastly improved. In the early days, insulin was obtained from cow and pig pancreases, which were plentiful. However, purification was extremely crude. Later, this insulin became much safer through techniques to eliminate contaminants.

Modern genetic engineering now allows the synthesis of human insulin identical to that found in the human body. This provides the insulin-treated diabetic population with a greatly improved source.

The major advantage of human insulin over the older beef and pork insulin is the elimination of allergic symptoms and irritation or allergic reactions at the injection site. Also, in some cases people become resistant to beef and pork insulins. Because human insulin matches naturally occurring insulin, is very pure, and doesn't cause allergic reactions; it is the preferred insulin at this time.

Insulin Attitude

Why is it that sometimes minor irritations become major aggravations? The paper cut when we stick our hand quickly into a file cabinet; the unnoticed staple left on the floor that finds our big toe as we walk across the carpet barefoot; the tiny prick of a straight pin as we remove it from a new dress or shirt—these can be painful for days. Why is this? Certainly it is no major trauma to this wondrous machine we call our human bodies. Usually it is mental aggravation that manifests as a nagging pain. It almost seems to throb as we dwell upon it.

However, your mind-set when you give yourself an insulin injection is diametrically opposed to these examples. The insulin injection is, after all, a planned event. It is no surprise. It's delivered into clean skin under the safest of conditions and therefore takes no bacteria into the tissue with it.

And you say the first time you gave yourself an insulin injection it was terribly painful? To this I just have to say, "Bunk!" True, your injection technique will improve, but even an awkward insulin injection is just not that big a deal. The injection itself takes less than ten seconds. And we are not getting a red-hot poker, merely a super-sharp, micro-fine stainless steel needle that has been developed with space-age technology. The disposable syringe industry is a science unto itself.

Today's Insulin Syringe

I use at least 1,000 insulin syringes each year. Multiply that number by the approximately 6 million insulin-using diabetics in this country alone and the numbers become staggering. Tens of thousands more insulin syringes are used in hospitals across the United States, and each one must be carefully manufactured under the highest quality control.

Take a good look at your insulin syringe. Note the snug fit of the plunger, the unit demarcations along the barrel, and the placement of the micro-fine needle at the end of the syringe. Become "user friendly" with the instruments you will use daily, possibly for the rest of your life. Note the balance of the syringe and become adept in handling it. It takes practice to develop good technique.

The typical insulin syringe is a 100-unit measuring instrument. One hundred units is equal to one cubic centimeter (cc.) of fluid. One cc., or 100 units, is also equal to one milliliter of fluid. So, one-half cc. is equal to 50 units and so forth. This helps you set reference points on the amount of insulin you give yourself every day.

I give myself 30 units of intermediate-acting insulin in the morning and 10 units in the evening—40 units every day. Because this is nearly 50 units, or one-half cc., I can calculate how long a vial of intermediate-acting insulin should last me. There are 10 cc. in a vial of intermediate-acting insulin. If I use about one-half cc. per day, the insulin vial will last me approximately 20 days.

Imagine you are supposed to take 10 units of regular insulin and 20 units of intermediate-acting insulin for a total dose of 30 units. If you are distracted and take 20 units of regular and 10 units of intermediate-acting, you are in big trouble. Unless your blood sugar is extremely high, the large dose of regular short-acting insulin will send you into an insulin reaction in less than one hour. So always be very careful with insulin and always double-check yourself.

Careless measurement can result in either high blood glucose or an insulin reaction. Both must be avoided. Even a veteran diabetic can make an error on occasion. Yes, I refer to myself again. You'll see I have made almost every mistake in the book. I try to point these out so you can avoid them.

Injection Background

Imagine you were a diabetic in 1964. After testing your urine for glucose (an outdated test today, but there were no home blood glucose monitors in those days), it was time to take the insulin injection. Your glass insulin syringe and stainless steel reusable needles were kept in a glass jar filled with alcohol, usually with sterile gauze pads lining the bottom. And the glass syringes had to be sterilized at least once a week. The syringes were either U-40 or U-80 and were matched with either U-40 or U-80 insulin. This match was critical, and if the pharmacist gave you U-80 insulin when you were using a U-40 syringe, you had big problems.

First, you had to wash the glass syringe of the alcohol it was stored in, then attach the stainless steel needle. The bore of the stainless steel needle was large enough to run a fine wire through for cleaning. Today's micro-fine needles are painless in comparison with the large-bore stainless steel needles of 25 to 30 years ago. In fact, you could run today's micro-fine needle through the bore of the old stainless steel needles, with room to spare.

When the needles became dull or developed a barb, you were instructed to run the angled needle point over some fine sandpaper. Ouch. The plunger traveled easily within the glass syringe barrel, creating the possibility of errors in insulin dose. I remember dropping my just-filled glass syringe onto the tile floor of my bathroom. If I had not kept a spare syringe in a separate glass jar, I would have been in trouble that morning. As it was, I still had to sterilize the spare syringe before I could use it.

Disposable needles were not introduced until the late 1960s. This represented a quantum leap in the convenience and ease of daily insulin injections. Even so, I still used my glass syringe until disposable syringes became widely marketed. After that, life became much easier.

Chapter Nine

Painless Injections

IF your diabetes is newly diagnosed, you'll get used to hearing people say, "Oh, no, you will have to give yourself shots for the rest of your life." That can cast a pall, if you let it. But consider the statement carefully.

We all have to do lots of things for the rest of our lives. We eat, sleep, brush our teeth. Now you have a new lifestyle to deal with, and it must become routine. I don't think many people give a second thought to showering and getting dressed each morning. Similarly, daily insulin must become second nature, a normal part of your life.

Insulin is another of the non-negotiable aspects of diabetes, so don't allow well-meaning friends or family to view shots as a negative part of your life. Don't be hostile; they have your best interest at heart. But do promote positive thinking in yourself and the people close to you.

I realize this is not always possible. We all have bouts of depression, loss, sadness, grief, and the like, but I always stress the positive outlook. How would I respond to the statement, "Oh no, you will have to give yourself shots for the rest of your life?" How about this approach? "Yes, you are right. I will have to take insulin injections for the rest of my life. But, without these life-sustaining injections, there wouldn't be any 'rest of my life.'" Remember, as a person with diabetes, part of your mission in life can be to educate others about diabetes.

The Injection ABCs

Okay, so how do you give yourself the perfect insulin injection? Here is my personal technique, which you can modify to suit yourself. For over 30 years, I have given myself an average of two insulin injections per day. That's over 20,000 injections—a lot of holes. I have developed my technique so that each and every injection is painless.

Find someplace where you can sit comfortably, someplace spacious and clean. After you have checked your blood glucose, lay out the necessary items: a fresh insulin syringe, disposable alcohol swab, and insulin vial or vials.

1. **Open the alcohol swab and carefully clean the tops of your insulin vials.** This is critical even with a new vial of insulin, and must be done each time you remove insulin from the vial. The alcohol creates a sterile environment over the rubber membrane and prevents bacteria from entering the vial.

2. **Remove the syringe end caps that protect the needle and plunger.** Move the plunger up and down several times to make sure it works well. Pull the plunger back to approximately the dosage of insulin required for your injection.

3. **Insert the needle into the vial of insulin and push the plunger all the way to zero.** This adds adequate air to the vial, which makes it easier to withdraw the insulin.

4. **Turn the vial over and hold it in your left hand (if you are right-handed).** You are now holding the vial upside down with the syringe protruding from the rubber membrane.

5. **Grasp the insulin vial in your left hand with your index finger and thumb and use your right hand to pull the syringe plunger.** Make sure the inside of the syringe is wet—to prevent bubble formation—by withdrawing the amount of insulin and pushing it back into the vial several times. Get comfortable with this technique to withdraw the correct

amount of insulin without air bubbles sticking to the sides of the syringe.

6. **Pull the plunger down to the amount of insulin your doctor has advised you to take.**

Remember, if you are mixing two different insulins, add the short-acting dosage insulin first, then add the intermediate- or long-acting dosage in the same syringe. For example, if you take 8 units of regular insulin and 26 units of intermediate insulin, always draw the 8 units of regular insulin first, then stick the syringe into the intermediate vial and pull the plunger down to the amount of the total dosage—a total of 34 units on the syringe.

When mixing two different insulins, make sure you understand this procedure and know the correct amount of insulin you're taking from each vial. Also, be sure to remove any air bubbles from the syringe with the first insulin. When the two insulins have mixed together it's impossible to know which insulin to add to get back to your correct dosage. So, be sure your first insulin dose is correct and free of air bubbles, then add the second insulin.

If you have trouble here, you will quickly learn the reasons for adding adequate volumes of air to your insulin vials and making sure you pull your first insulin into the syringe several times to wet the barrel of the syringe. Patient practice is the name of the game. If you do get air bubbles in the syringe with your first insulin type, simply push the insulin back into the vial and then draw the correct dosage into the syringe again.

If an air bubble persists, remove the syringe from the vial and tap the upright syringe several times to move the bubble to the top of the syringe near the needle. Then push the plunger just slightly to push out the air bubble. Add more insulin if needed to arrive at your required dose. It is very important to pay meticulous attention to your insulin dose. If your doctor prescribes 10 units of regular insulin in the morning, he means just that, not 8 or 12.

Pain-Free Injection

With your correct insulin dose in the syringe, you are ready to inject. First, do you know why shots are sometimes painful? There are several reasons. With intramuscular (IM) injections (not used for insulin), the needle is long and can cause pain as it enters the muscle. More likely, the pain with an IM injection is caused by the thick drug being injected. Also, there are some particularly sensitive areas of the body that are painful no matter what size needle or type of drug is used. With diabetes, we can choose less tender sites.

An insulin injection is given subcutaneously—meaning just below the skin. So, why is it still painful? Well, here is a secret most diabetics and doctors forget: If you use an alcohol swab to clean an area for your injection site, be sure to let the alcohol dry before injecting. Most painful insulin injections happen when you give the injection immediately after the area is wiped with the wet alcohol. Ouch, that alcohol burns. It took me a long time to figure this out—and I want you to benefit from my experience.

So here are my tips for a pain-free injection:

1. **After you allow your injection site to dry, place the insulin syringe comfortably in your hand.** I like to place the syringe between my index and middle fingers at about the midway point of the syringe, thumb resting on top of the plunger. Place the heel of this hand just above the injection site. Rest your hand comfortably here as you place the needle of the syringe close to your skin.

2. **With just a slight fast forward motion, quickly insert the needle below the skin.**

3. **Using your thumb, press the plunger down to deliver your insulin.** The injection is over in a matter of seconds.

4. **Apply the alcohol swab to the injection site while the syringe is still in place with the plunger all the way down.** It is important to apply slight pressure at the injection site as you remove the needle from the site. This ensures that

the insulin stays inside and does not travel up and out as you remove the needle.

5. **Gently rub the injection site with the alcohol swab for several minutes.** In the old days we were advised not to rub at all, but recent research has shown that gently rubbing the injection site distributes the insulin and may promote better absorption.

Remember, your injection technique will improve with experience. Have patience, and make your goal the quintessential painless insulin injection. I've done it, and you can, too.

You may also want to try the newer devices that make giving an injection easier. Some accelerate needle insertion into the skin. Others create portals into which you inject insulin, thus minimizing needle punctures. (See Chapter 10 for more information on injection aids.)

Selecting Sites

It is very important to rotate your insulin injection sites. What are the best sites? Recent research shows that much better control can be achieved if you give insulin in the abdomen. The lower and more consistent blood glucose readings are good enough evidence for me to use this area often. Talk with your health care team about the best injection site for you and rotate within that site.

The abdomen is also a convenient site when you are going out to dinner or to a social gathering. Many times I have taken my insulin injection at a crowded restaurant in plain view of everyone at the table. I have accomplished this so quickly and unobtrusively that no one even notices. It requires just a slight opening of the shirt or blouse. Over the years I have encountered one problem with this injection area. With too many repeat injections, you may find a build-up of fatty tissue that produces fatty mounds. This build-up can be difficult to break down even with exercise, so don't rely on this area for continued use.

Try not to overuse any injection site. The upper arms, one inch or so below the shoulder, are good sites. They usually have lots of soft fatty tissue to easily inject into. Don't inject much farther down than two or three inches from the shoulder.

Many people use the thighs and buttocks as injection sites. The upper thighs have a large surface area and are generally good for injections. The outer thighs and farther around to the back portion of the upper thigh area are best. The inner thigh area is sensitive, and it's easy to break down delicate tissue in that area. Avoid overuse of the top portion of the thighs. This can also become sensitive, and overuse may produce tissue buildup similar to what I described for the abdomen.

The buttocks is a good surface area for injections. The first time I tried this, I had had diabetes for just six months. I was using a glass syringe with a glass plunger that had to be held against the barrel of the syringe to prevent the plunger from slipping and losing the insulin. The needle was a large stainless-steel reusable instrument.

This needle was new, so I guess I should be thankful for small favors. I reached back around to give myself the injection. With my left hand, I pinched some tissue, and with my right hand I nervously jammed the needle home. Well, not exactly. The needle went directly into the inner fleshy part of my thumb. This was not a quintessential painless insulin injection. The thumb has many veins and nerves, and I gave myself a jolt of red hot pain.

It may be difficult to try a new area when you are comfortable using a particular spot, but keep in mind that after you get used to a new spot, it will no longer be intimidating. And thumbs are definitely not on the diabetic's authorized list of insulin injection sites.

Chapter Ten

Insulin
Delivery Systems

THE syringe is the most common insulin-delivery system because it is easy to use and convenient. (Jet injection systems and insulin pumps, which will be discussed in this chapter, are also options for some diabetics.)

Through the years I've given myself shots in some unusual settings: in the cabin of a Lear jet, driving a red Ferrari with the top down, and in a rather unclean bathroom in Mexico. I can't count how many times I've given myself a shot on a commercial flight. I'd almost always get strange looks as I undid the lower button of my shirt and jabbed myself in the abdomen. I've taken syringes with me from classroom to emergency room, and from research lab to restaurant—practically everywhere.

I'll never forget the time I was traveling back to the mainland from Hawaii in the late 1960s. This was a time of hippies, anti-war demonstrations, and drugs, drugs, and more drugs. As I walked through customs at Honolulu International Airport, the inspector gave me a long look. He saw a 19-year-old surfer with long hair, a tan face, and salt-water surfer eyes. He asked to look inside my suitcase. I didn't have anything to hide so I was happy to comply. "Do you have any weed, speed, or seed, son?" "No sir," I said. Just then he opened my suitcase and found a package of 100 syringes. He didn't say a word. He just smiled and waved me on. I can only guess the large number of syringes in plain sight told him I had diabetes.

If he had asked why I had so many syringes, I could have shown my diabetes identification card and insulin prescriptions. I suggest you carry a diabetes identification card with you at all times, especially while traveling. It lists your name, address, phone number, physician, and emergency symptoms for people unfamiliar with diabetes. Identification bracelets and neck chains are also available. More information is available from the American Diabetes Association or your doctor.

Repeat Usage

Although disposable insulin syringes are designed to be used just once, you can reuse them for up to a week and save some money. But, you must remember to use a good sterile technique.

Of course, a limiting factor to the life of the syringe is the sharpness of the needle. If the needle is dull, don't reuse it. Typically, I will use the same syringe for a week—two injections per day—and then start with a fresh syringe. Even if you reuse a syringe only once, you will save some money. I repeat, however, you should not reuse a syringe until you have completely mastered a good sterile technique.

Injection Aids

A variation on the everyday syringe is the pen-like syringe. These pen devices hold pre-filled cartridges of insulin and can quickly inject small amounts of insulin. Many people prefer their size and convenience over the larger standard syringes.

Many diabetics have also come to appreciate other types of injection aids. Several devices help accelerate needle insertion into the skin by using a spring-loaded syringe holder. Subcutaneous infusion sets are also available. With these, a catheter remains beneath the skin for several days. Insulin is injected through an external port, minimizing the number of needle punctures.

Another injection system has no needle. Yes, you read correctly: No needle. Insulin penetrates the skin through a high-pressure air blast. The military tested air-jet injection systems back in the early 1960s in mass inoculations of military personnel and their families. I know because I was one of those who waited in line to get a shot. Most of us kids didn't know whether to cry because the air blast was uncomfortable or to be happy because there were no hideous looking needles to be stabbed into our arms.

Although there is no needle, an air-jet injection still penetrates the skin, causing some pain. The more proficient you are in your technique—needle or jet injection—the less pain you will feel.

Jet injection systems are not for everyone. People who should not use jet injectors include those who have bleeding disorders, such as hemophilia; are very thin; have little or no strength in their hands; or have arthritis of the hands or wrists.

Poor vision or blindness can make the use of a jet injector challenging, but at least one model has features helpful for the visually impaired. I decided to try a jet injector after I became blind in 1985—to prove to myself I could use an instrument originally designed for the sighted diabetic. I attended a training course at a hospital and persevered in the use of the jet injector.

Instrument Characteristics

Using a jet injection system requires attention to detail and a willingness to develop and learn a new technique. Once the jet injector is loaded with your insulin dose, place it firmly against your skin at the chosen site and simply press the discharge button at the top of the instrument. Because it is easy to use, you can inject sites you can't reach with a syringe.

Some jet injection systems use disposable "nozzles" so

cleaning and sterilization is not needed. Other systems must be thoroughly cleaned every two weeks because insulin tends to stick to the components. The separated parts should be sterilized in boiling water for at least 20 minutes. If the system is not used every day, it must be cleaned more often. Blood glucose should be checked at least once a day when using the jet injection system. I suggest checking it two or three times a day.

After many years of injections with a syringe, the absorption rate of insulin can slow down in those injected tissue areas, preventing the even spread of insulin. This so-called "pooling" can delay the onset of insulin. Jet injectors blast insulin into the site in a uniform pattern, increasing its absorption. This is thought to be easier on the tissue, which is especially important for children because it helps to minimize damage to the delicate fat layer beneath the skin.

It has been reported that use of a jet injector tends to reduce insulin antibody formation. Insulin antibodies tend to cause a resistance to the uptake of insulin at the cellular level, creating the need for additional insulin, which in turn creates more insulin resistance. Use of the jet injection system may help achieve better diabetic control.

Another possible benefit of jet injection is patient compliance. Some people are more willing to take their insulin when they don't have to use a needle.

The Insulin Pump

The insulin pump is a marvel of high-tech ingenuity and design. It is about the size of a phone beeper and worn outside of the body. A computerized pump sends a steady, measured amount of insulin through a cannula (a small plastic tube) with a small needle that is placed into fatty tissue and held with tape. This needle must be changed and moved to another infusion site every one to three days. In newer products, the needle is removed and a catheter remains in place. It must be refilled with insulin every one or two days.

Insulin is delivered by the pump in two different modes. The basal dose is released as a steady amount throughout the day. This rate is determined by you and your doctor, based on your level of exercise, activity, and food intake. A different basal rate can be set for each hour of the day depending on your needs. If you find that your blood glucose is high or you're about to eat, a bolus dose can be administered. For example, with each press of a button on the pump, a bolus dose of 0.5 units of insulin is delivered.

The pump uses short-acting insulin because it provides a better control system. Imagine yourself connected to a small instrument carrying life-sustaining insulin. You will sleep with this pump, eat with it, work with it—everything you normally do in life. Currently available pumps are water resistant or waterproof, though cases are available. Still, you may remove the pump while you shower, swim, or partici- pate in other activities. But most of the time you will remain attached to it. The pump should be worn on a belt or carried in a pocket or some other convenient location where you can program and monitor it. Newer pumps sound alarms to signal dangerous conditions such as a blocked tube or low supply of insulin.

The insulin pump has many benefits. Most importantly, it closely mimics the pancreas by delivering small doses of insulin throughout the day. Another advantage is you are con- nected to the pump all day. This helps many people avoid the convenient denial of diabetes, something that happens only too frequently with us diabetics.

For all the benefits of insulin pumps, they are expensive (costing as much as $5000) and do demand an above-average desire to control diabetes. Furthermore, insulin pumps do not sense your need for insulin. You still need to monitor blood glucose levels—at least four to six times per day. Even so, in my opinion, this is a definite benefit, not an inconvenience. You are acutely aware of your blood glucose at different times of the day and, therefore, in better control.

If you want maximum control and are willing to make the commitment to strict diabetes management skills, then the pump is something you should investigate with your doctor. Currently, I do not use an insulin pump. I planned to use one in 1984, just before I lost my eyesight. However, some blind diabetics do use the insulin pump.

Implantable Pumps

Since the early 1970s, researchers have been working on an implantable insulin pump. Surgically placed under the skin in the abdomen area, the pump releases insulin as programmed by remote unit, similar to a television remote control. The pump needs to be filled approximately monthly by injecting insulin a membrane-covered reservoir on the pump. It's almost like an artificial pancreas, though blood glucose must still be checked.

An implantable insulin pump is approved for use in Europe, but at this time, it has not received approval by the United States Food and Drug Administration (FDA).

Nasal Inhalation

Taking insulin through the nose—much like inhaling an antihistamine—has been studied for many years. It would eliminate many of the shots that some people fear. However, syringes would still be used in a secondary role. Unfortunately, nasal inhalation of insulin has proved unsatisfactory, for many reasons.

The most important problem is maintaining correct dosages. Also, researchers don't know if long-term inhalation of insulin will cause sinus problems. Studies continue throughout the world.

There are many things to consider when choosing an insulin delivery system. One that is right for me, after more than 30 years of diabetes, may not be right for you. Take a close look at each system with your doctor and find one that is good for you. And be sure to always talk with your doctor or diabetes management team about your concerns.

Chapter Eleven

Current Theory and Treatment

THE knowledge and treatment of diabetes have vastly changed over the years. Compare the disposable syringe to the old glass syringes and the compact and sensitive glucose monitors to the clumsy method of urine glucose testing used just three to four decades ago. Think of the great strides in the purification of insulin and the sophisticated DNA technology now used to make human insulin.

Still, while we're amazed at the developments in diabetes management, we must remember that a cure seems as far away as ever. For now, diabetes is an incurable disease with far-reaching ramifications. Insulin is only a management tool; it is not a cure. All the devices to manage diabetes, including this book and others, are just tools. Your knowledge is important in the effective management of diabetes. Your doctor and diabetes educator play a necessary role, too.

Making Healthy Choices

When you look for a doctor to guide your management program, remember not all doctors are knowledgeable and experienced in treating diabetes. Most general practitioners and family practice doctors do have a basic understanding of diabetes management. Find a doctor who is not only a good diagnostician and clinician, but also a good teacher and, most importantly, a good learner and listener. Then work with your doctor and do your best to comply with his or her recommendations.

Doctors have long recognized the importance of compliance as illustrated in this story about a friend when he was in medical school:

One of the tough, old internal medicine professors asked his class, "What is the biggest problem in diabetes?" Of course, there are many problems in diabetes. After two students answered incorrectly, my friend raised his hand and sheepishly said, "Patient compliance?"

The professor was amazed and delighted my friend had answered this rather tricky question. Puzzled, the professor said, "Wait a second. Did I have your brother in this class some years ago?"

"No, sir," replied the student. Still, the professor was surprised this young student could get the answer right. When pressed, my friend finally admitted his father had been a student under the old professor and had passed down the lesson. My friend received an 'A' in the class.

Problems with compliance do go back a long way. Most doctors will tell you getting a patient to follow their advice can be difficult and frustrating. Some patients don't listen or believe the consequences. Doctors can advise until they are blue in the face that smoking is fatalistic and stupid. But if the patient doesn't quit, there is nothing the doctor can do but watch the tobacco take its toll. If your doctor insists you monitor your blood glucose three times a day, and you don't, who are you hurting?

For the best care, give your doctor lots of information about yourself. A doctor can better evaluate your daily routine if you keep a log of blood glucose levels, noting reaction times and even instances of overeating or having a sweet. This is so much better than the diabetic who, when asked how his blood glucose is running, answers, "Just fine." If the doctor has to pry information from you, both of you will most likely become frustrated.

Treatment

When I was first diagnosed with diabetes, I was told to give myself one shot a day of a mixture of short-acting regular insulin and intermediate-acting insulin.

A few years later, doctors began advising the two-shot-per-day program. In this method, an additional injection of insulin is given before the evening meal, usually in a much smaller amount than the morning injection. Many people today are using the two-injection regimen.

In the mid-1980s, the four-injection method became popular in maintaining tight blood glucose control. At the time, many of us suspected tight control would delay or prevent complications. But, as mentioned throughout this book, we didn't have the proof until the DCCT. (For the DCCT, intensive control involved three or four daily injections of insulin or the use of an insulin pump. Importantly, it also meant frequent blood glucose monitoring and adjustments in insulin to match exercise and food intake.) With all of this evidence that strict control of your diabetes can prevent complications, do you feel lucky enough to ignore it? I don't.

Commonly, with a four-shot method, an injection of regular insulin is given before every meal and intermediate- or long-acting at bedtime. Because the short-acting insulin peaks relatively quickly, blood glucose must be carefully checked to guard against hypo- and hyperglycemia. You need to check your blood glucose at least once every six hours.

A commitment to careful management is a must if you choose an intensive treatment method. For one thing, intensive treatment—with its more frequent injections, blood tests, and doctor's visits—is double the cost of conventional treatment. Secondly, it means paying more attention to your diabetes than you might have thought possible. Each day you must make time to perform several blood glucose tests and insulin injections. You also must guard against common risks of tight blood glucose control such as insulin reactions and weight gain.

Clearly, tight control is not for everyone. Your lifestyle and your personal commitment to diabetes are important in deciding the best treatment method for you. I've used the two-injection method for many years and have tight control of my blood glucose. For me, the four-shot method is not appropriate; it would be difficult without eyesight.

An intensive treatment program with multiple injections is also not recommended for elderly people or children under the age of 7. Moreover, intensive therapy can be unsafe for people with certain health conditions including coronary heart disease, irregular heart beats, and other types of heart disease. People more susceptible to hypoglycemia are also cautioned.

One of the keys to successful diabetic control, no matter what method you choose, is to rely on the expertise and support of your diabetes team. Endocrinologists, certified diabetes educators, dietitians, and other health professionals understand the issues you face. They also know the latest management techniques and equipment that lead to a higher quality of life.

Preventing Diabetes

The theory of what causes diabetes has changed over the years. When I was first diagnosed, doctors looked closely for a genetic link. Over the years, scientists have unsuccessfully searched for viruses that may cause diabetes.

Now, most doctors think the body, for unknown reasons, destroys the insulin-producing cells within the pancreas. If this sounds improbable, consider what happens when proliferative retinopathy and neovascularization affect the eye; it destroys itself.

The prevention of diabetes, both Type 1 and Type 2, is receiving lots of attention and research dollars. Already underway is the Diabetes Prevention Trial—Type 1 (DPT-1), which is studying the immediate family members of those with Type 1 diabetes. Family members have a 15-fold higher risk of developing Type 1 diabetes than the general population. The nationwide study, which is slated to end in the year 2002, is testing whether daily insulin injections or oral insulin will prevent diabetes.

For Type 2 diabetes, a similar study is in the works called the Diabetes Prevention Program (DPP). This six-year study is examining at-risk individuals and whether Type 2 diabetes can be prevented or delayed by lowering blood glucose levels through diet and exercise or medication.

Chapter Twelve

Meal Planning Guidelines

F OOD has always been a major focus in diabetes management. Not long ago, the attention was on what foods were off-limits to all diabetics. Fortunately, we now realize that we can eat most foods, as long as they are part of a meal plan based on each individual's needs and overall health.

When I was 15 and a newly diagnosed diabetic in the early 1960s, diabetes manuals listed column after column of restricted foods. I even made a game of reciting the long list of restricted items. Of course, everything with sugar was either restricted entirely or limited to minute quantities.

While in the hospital getting regulated to my insulin requirements, the typical lunch and dinner was an onion salad. That's right, sliced onions and vinegar. To this day the memory produces a cold sweat. For breakfast, they served powdered eggs cooked without a hint of butter, limp white toast, skim milk, and if I was lucky, a strip or two of bacon that had been sacrificed to the fire gods.

When I returned home, the American Diabetes Association's exchange lists for meal planning became my guide. (The six exchange lists group foods that are similar in carbohydrate, protein, fat, and calories when you choose them in the amounts listed.) For every meal, my mother carefully weighed and measured each food item. She even bought small metal bowls that held the correct amount of vegetables and meat I was allowed.

After several years, I felt I was still in the hospital getting meals from the hospital kitchen. My metal bowls with weighed-out food stood out against the family dinnerware.

Finally, as I sat down one evening to another clinical dinner, I lashed out. Not at my loving mother, but at the institutional setting of my meal. The family agreed I would eat just like them, with no special bowls. My food was still measured, but it was put on a plate like the rest of the family.

An Individualized Meal Plan

If you have never been on a meal plan, it may be intimidating. You may even think of it as restrictive. On the contrary, today's specialized meal plans are planned by a doctor or dietitian and targeted for your diabetes. A meal plan—plus insulin or oral medications, glucose monitoring, and exercise—are essential components of an effective diabetes management program.

A dietitian can help you learn different ways to plan your meals and snacks. Counting food exchanges or carbohydrates are two of the most popular approaches. Not only do you learn which healthy foods to eat and how much, but also how to match meals and insulin action times. And the new meal plan isn't designed for just today or next month. It's a guide for the rest of your life.

The newest nutrition recommendations from the American Diabetes Association (ADA) do not suggest a single way to eat. The proportions of carbohydrates, protein, and fat in your meal plan depend on your specific situation and health needs. In general, though, the ADA recommendations are similar to those for everyone, diabetic or not: Eat a variety of foods that are low in fat and high in complex carbohydrates (they provide the most nutrients per calorie).

Specifically, if you do not have signs of kidney disease,

between 10 and 20 percent of calories should come from protein. If you develop kidney disease, a maximum protein intake of 0.8 gram of protein per kilogram of body weight per day is recommended. The ADA also recommends that no more than 10 percent of your calories come from saturated fat, and limits cholesterol intake to less than 300 milligrams per day. Each day, you should strive to consume 20 to 35 grams of fiber and no more than 2,400 to 3,000 milligrams of sodium.

Sugar's role in diabetes has long been explored. Today, not only do we know that sugar does not cause diabetes, but research also shows that sugars and starches have similar effects on blood glucose levels. That means the amount of carbohydrate, not the source, is the issue. Moderate amounts of sugar can be a part of a well-balanced diabetic meal plan, the ADA says. Even so, as I discuss later in this chapter, you should not go overboard with sweets.

A Healthier World

Why doesn't everyone follow a healthy diet? Because most Americans have become slaves to convenience, fast foods, high salt, high sugar, little exercise, and sitting in front of the television. But many are starting to realize the health problems of high fat and cholesterol, which the diabetic meal plan has always stressed to avoid.

I wonder what it would be like if everyone was on a diabetic meal plan. Would there be fewer instances of heart attack, hypertension, strokes, atherosclerosis, and arteriosclerosis? Would there be fewer hyperactive children because they would avoid sugar-loaded cereals, sodas, and snacks? You are now embarking on a meal plan everyone should follow. And it's not just for diabetes management. It is a vigorous meal plan designed to improve your cardiovascular system, nerve transmission, and energy level—and to prolong your life.

The diabetic meal plan requires education, good management skills, and a common sense approach to eating well. The worst thing you can do is ignore your meal plan. Diabetes requires constant attention. I know this isn't easy. But it must be done. Eating the correct amount of food is a special challenge.

Overeating

Eat more food than necessary, and guess what? You got it: high blood glucose.

Most food has some form of sugar in it. So even if you skip dessert and don't add sugar to your coffee after a large meal, you may still have high blood glucose. If the meal has more calories than you were entitled to on your meal plan, your insulin will not control the extra calories. The excess will spill over into the blood and create high blood glucose.

So eating the proper amount of food at every meal is important, not only to avoid high blood glucose, but also to avoid low blood glucose.

This point is confusing to some people. However, if you will be strenuously exercising or under some stress that requires high energy, you may eat a little more food than called for. That energy we need comes from carbohydrates, which are found in sugar, starch, and fiber.

I can imagine what you may be thinking now: "A lot of great philosophy, but what's done on a daily basis?" You must consult your doctor or dietitian for your particular meal plan needs. However, here is what I do, and why.

Fiber

Fiber occurs naturally in many vegetables, fruits, and in grains such as oats and bran. I'm a strong advocate of fiber in the diet. The reason is simple.

Diabetes tends to cause the formation of deposits, primarily made of cholesterol and fat, on the inner surface of important arteries. As more material is deposited, the artery narrows and hardens. This reduces blood flow, and therefore oxygen, to areas such as the heart, brain, kidney, and retina.

However, if we eat a diet high in fiber, the buildup of cholesterol and fatty deposits in blood vessels is reduced. Think of fiber as tiny brooms that sweep out the fatty deposits, clearing the way for increased blood flow and oxygen. Significantly reducing the amount of cholesterol and fat in the diet also can help prevent the deposits from forming in the first place.

There are two forms of fiber: soluble and insoluble. Soluble fiber completely dissolves in solution, much like salt disappearing in a glass of water. High amounts of soluble fiber are found in oat bran, legumes (dried beans and peas), barley, and some fruits and vegetables. Insoluble fiber does not completely dissolve in water. Good sources of insoluble fiber are wheat bran, whole wheat or grains, and some vegetables.

Fiber is not digested or absorbed in the bloodstream. What goes in through the mouth goes out with a bowel movement. The important actions of fiber occur entirely in the gut. Soluble fiber is especially useful for diabetics because it mixes with fluid in the gut to form a gel-like lining on the gut. This decreases the ability of the gut to absorb fat. Therefore a small percentage passes though the gut without being absorbed.

Soluble fiber also appears to surround the bile molecules secreted by the liver. This prevents the bile from being reabsorbed by the gut. The bile then passes through the gut and is excreted in the feces. What is the liver's response? It removes cholesterol from the blood to make more bile.

Soluble fiber has another benefit for diabetics. The gel that coats the lining of the gut also slows the absorption of glucose. Because glucose is absorbed slower, blood glucose levels don't peak so high. If consumed consistently in high quantities, soluble fiber tends to reduce daily insulin needs.

You won't get enough fiber if your diet consists of strictly meat and potatoes (although potatoes do have some fiber). You should try to increase dietary fiber, even if it means taking a supplement. Fiber supplements are easy to take in the evening along with your late-night snack. Of course, with any significant diet change, you should consult your doctor and continue to closely monitor your blood sugar.

Vegetables

Fiber increases the level of high-density lipoproteins (HDL cholesterol), the good guys, and decreases low-density lipoproteins (LDL cholesterol), the bad guys. We should eat more leafy vegetables because they are high in fiber. You already eat plenty? Then try to eat more. Salads made of leaf lettuce, cucumbers, tomatoes, and onions are especially good. They contain few calories and can be eaten in large quantities. I especially like cabbage, cauliflower, and broccoli salads by themselves, or combined as super salads.

When it comes to salads, I make a ritual of it. I make sure my vegetables are clean and my knives are sharp and easy to use. I like to eat organically grown vegetables as much as possible. They are grown without chemicals and are better for you.

But watch out. Salads become heavy with calories when you add salad dressing. Remember, most salad dressings at restaurants are made with fattening cheeses and rich sour creams and oils. Limit the amount of salad dressing. It's supposed to dress a salad, not drown it.

Water

I enjoy drinking water, and I drink more of it than most people. Plenty of water keeps the system flushed of impurities, which is especially good for the kidneys of diabetics. Every time you pass a water cooler or fountain, take a drink. At meal times, keep your water glass full.

Breakfast

A healthy breakfast is important because you must take insulin to start the day.

Eggs and bacon every morning, however, are not healthy. So they're out. You certainly can't eat them every day and maintain a low cholesterol and blood fat level. Egg yolks are rich in cholesterol and bacon is high in fat and salt. Try to limit yourself to two egg yolks a week at the most.

Milk is good, but remember, whole milk contains fat and cholesterol. A high fiber cereal with skim milk is a good breakfast. Add an apple or banana and your breakfast is even better. Fruit juices should be limited, however, because of their natural sugar.

Are you tired of the same old breakfast? Your meal plan may allow some wheat-grain toast with crunchy peanut butter and a little honey or jelly. Add half an apple and a glass of skim milk for a nice breakfast. Be creative. Try a piece of wheat-grain toast with some low-fat cheese and a slice of tomato on top; broil it for a few minutes. This is great with a cup of coffee, a glass of skim milk, and an apple. Check your meal plan to see if you can have several pieces of toast prepared this way.

Lunch

Lunch is important too, but it's best to stay away from fast food restaurants. Most meals at the fast food places are for taste, and until just recently, were not for the diet-restricted person at all. Now they're doing a better job and even offer nutrition fact sheets. Keep in mind a heavy, greasy meal at lunch time can slow you down during the latter part of the day and make it difficult to accomplish anything.

A tuna-fish salad with mixed greens, a tuna-fish salad sandwich, or a chicken salad sandwich with soup are all good luncheon ideas. Try to include a garden salad with your lunch. If you must eat at a fast food restaurant, avoid the double meat, double bacon, sourdough burger. It may taste delicious, but it may also contain as many calories as you are allowed for an entire day, and may have twice the amount of fat and salt you need for an entire week.

Dinner

Do you have a steak or a fancy chicken breast every dinner? You shouldn't. Instead, try a big garden salad mixed with salmon, tuna, or chicken. Add fruit and wheat crackers and you have an excellent meal. Watch the amount of salad dressing you add. You can make your own by using herbs and spices with olive oil and wine vinegar.

It's fine to eat a juicy steak once in a while. But red meat contains a large amount of fat and must be watched closely. Always trim off the excess fat. My rule of thumb is to eat red meat no larger than the size of a deck of cards. I still eat red meat for a balanced diet, but I eat much less than I used to. I've replaced most of it with chicken and fish. Remember, though, all animal foods contain some cholesterol.

Cranberry juice is a good option to the usual beverages at meals. It helps to flush the kidneys, and, although it contains sugar, is good to drink regularly.

Snacks

Have a late-night snack before you go to sleep—perhaps a piece of cheese and some crackers, a glass of skim milk, and a small piece of fruit. Your dietitian can tell you how much you should eat each night. Sometimes I replace the cheese with a slice of chicken or ham. Try a little cream cheese on crackers for something different. Be careful, though. I've been known to get carried away and eat half a box of crackers and a lot of cream cheese. Hey, this is a snack, after all, not a main course. (Yes, my blood glucose was high in the morning.)

I suggest you obtain one of the excellent cookbooks on the market for people with diabetes. This book can't contain all the recipes and information on meal planning, but I want to get you started on becoming food-conscious. Don't feel like a prisoner who eats only bread and water. On the other hand, you can't feast on everything that comes before you.

Changing (Sweet) Taboos

Most people think sweets are off limits to people with diabetes. They don't think we can eat anything "fun." This is simply not true.

Diabetic meal plans are created for today's society and adaptable to most situations. Yes, you may have a piece of cake, some sugar soda, or a piece of chocolate candy at the birthday party. BUT (and this is the kicker) you must be very careful about eating too much of these once totally taboo items. You may eat a small piece of cherry pie if you substitute it for another food in your meal plan, but you should not eat a giant slice or two.

Even though sweets are not forbidden, it's best to avoid them. The occasional sweet will probably do no harm, but you shouldn't think it's OK to eat all you want. Calorie-free sugar substitutes, on the other hand, do not raise blood glucose levels because they do not contain carbohydrates.

If you don't totally deny yourself an occasional sweet, you shouldn't feel deprived. A strict denial program may increase the desire to eat sweets. This may lead to feelings of guilt and resentment—in which you feel you are the only one in the world who has to give up so much. To compensate, you may stray further and further from the correct meal plan.

Allow your mind to enjoy the thought of a sweet snack once in a while, rather than dwelling on never being able to enjoy these items again.

Portable Rations

Driving can be stressful and physically demanding at times. Sometimes you get stuck in traffic jams. Other times wild drivers speed by or cut you off. We should always have a supply of candy, orange juice, and cheese and crackers—if not sandwiches—should the worst happen.

You never know. What if you have an insulin reaction? With emergency rations in the car, you avoid potential danger. In fact, you should keep a "care package" with you everywhere.

I've used my care package more times than I ever imagined. It includes: three boxes of orange juice; three packages of crackers and peanut butter; one bag of individually wrapped hard candy; two packages of glucose gel; and syringes, extra insulin, and alcohol pads.

Alcohol: A Case Study

What about drinking alcohol? The following case history reveals my position:

A 36-year-old man in good health, with diabetes for over 20 years, attended a party that lasted from 8 p.m. to midnight. During the evening, he had four drinks of Scotch whiskey and diet Seven-up. The man was active, dancing, and talking to friends. Because he ate several sandwiches and snacks at the party, he skipped his usual snack before going to bed at 1 a.m.

The whiskey, which usually acts to lower blood glucose, did just that. Between 4 and 5 a.m., he started to have an insulin reaction. Normally he would have awakened, but the alcohol had dulled his senses. He went deeper into the low blood glucose state until his father heard him convulsing at 5:30 a.m.

The local doctor was called. The diabetic's teeth were so tightly clenched there was no way to give orange juice or candy by mouth. The violent convulsions continued until an infusion of 60 grams of glucose took effect. His measured blood glucose level was 23 mg/dl (1.3 mmol/L). Normal blood glucose levels are between 70 and 110 mg/dl (3.9 and 6.1 mmol/L).

What happened here? This diabetic was used to waking up during late night and early morning insulin reactions. But this time, the diabetic's body was numbed by the alcohol and he slept through it.

Now, do I suggest you drink alcohol? I was the man in this story. Still, this is a difficult issue. I believe alcohol should be kept to an absolute minimum, but a glass of wine with dinner may help with digestion. You are allowed to deduct fat exchanges on your meal plan to compensate for beer. You may give up fruit exchanges to have a glass of wine. If you do drink alcohol, remember you're taking a risk.

Chapter Thirteen

Exercise Guidelines

EXERCISE is the third key part of diabetes management, along with insulin or oral medications and meal planning. I've been an advocate of vigorous exercise programs for a long time. In my youth, I earned a black belt in Japanese karate. I pushed myself while surfing in Hawaii as a college student and never suffered an insulin reaction in the water. Later, I played tennis and racquetball. Although I was never good at either sport, I benefited from the exercise. I also enjoyed high school basketball and baseball.

Exercise, in any form, is extremely important because it controls blood glucose. Vigorous exercise can reduce moderately high levels of blood glucose, thereby controlling diabetes without extra insulin.

Before you begin a fitness program, talk with your doctor about any health problems that may keep you from exercising safely. Extremely high or low blood glucose levels, heart disease, retinopathy, and other conditions may limit your activity choices or necessitate certain precautions.

Insulin, diet, and exercise must be balanced for good diabetic control. Your activities may change the amount of insulin you need. If you exercise a lot, perhaps you'll have to reduce your insulin to avoid insulin reactions. If you stop exercising without changing your insulin amount or reducing your diet, you will end up with high blood glucose levels. If you take more insulin to manage the high glucose levels, then you risk gaining weight. Consult your doctor for an exercise program and appropriate insulin levels.

The Exercise of Choice

Of all the types of exercise, aerobic exercise, done on a regular basis, is one of the most beneficial because it strengthens the heart and circulatory system. Many people think aerobic exercise only is possible in an aerobics dance class with pumping music. Actually, any movement that gets your heart pumping and makes you breathe deeper qualifies as an aerobic activity.

It's fine if you don't like participating in sports or going to an exercise club. Exercise experts say a walking program is better for your cardiovascular system than nearly anything else. Walking may even be better than jogging because it's easier on the joints.

This is especially encouraging for me because my blindness restricts me from most sports, although I still train in karate. I enjoy taking a long walk in the evening, usually with my mother and father or a friend, and sharing a pleasant conversation. Thirty minutes passes in a flash. The important thing to remember with a walking program is you must walk long enough and briskly enough to produce a good cardiovascular workout.

Remember to check with your doctor before starting an exercise program. Also, check your blood glucose frequently and be prepared with a "care package" of sweets, including items such as orange juice and hard candy.

Simple Exercises

Upside-down butterfly: Lie flat on your back on the floor. With arms at your sides, raise your legs about 12 inches in the air. Lower and raise them in counts of five. Breathe in through the nose for the full count. Breathe out through the mouth with the next count of five. Work your way up to a count of 100.

Ups and downs: Ever notice how much time we spend in the bathroom? Use this time for some exercise. While shaving or drying your hair, raise up and down on your toes for a count of 100. Do these slowly to get maximum effect in the toes, feet, and calf muscles.

Rock stomach: While shaving or drying your hair, take a deep breath through your nose. Hold it in and tighten your stomach muscles for a count of 20. Do as many repetitions as time allows.

Steering wheel crush: When you're in the car with nothing to do but listen to the stereo, try some dynamic muscle tension. Grab the steering wheel and push inward with both hands. Tighten your stomach muscles and add force from the inner arms to the shoulders.

Coffee break escape: While your coworkers stand around the coffee pot at break time, take a brisk walk around the building. On your way back, get that cup of coffee and drink it at your desk. It pays to be enterprising.

Desk lift: If you work at a desk or counter, place both hands under it and lift as if to raise the desk toward the ceiling. Tighten your stomach muscles at the same time.

Leg stretch: If your work is sedentary, stretch your legs for a count of 20 every hour or so. Release and relax completely. This will increase circulation in the legs if done regularly. Make sure your office chair doesn't have a ridge at the edge that restricts your legs. If it does, ask for another chair.

Don't forget to breathe: Whenever you think of it, try to take a deep breath through the nose and hold it for as long as you can. Expel completely through the mouth. Repeat a few times and notice the renewed feeling. Many times we are so stressed out, we simply forget to breathe deeply.

Crow's neck stretch: Turn your head as far to the left as you can. Then stretch it a bit farther to the left. Do the same to the right. Repeat this several times to loosen the neck muscles and relieve strain.

Twist and shout: While standing, stretch your arms out in front with your hands together. Twist the upper body and arms while keeping the legs together, feet pointed ahead. The shout is optional but sure does relieve a lot of built-up stress!

This isn't an exhaustive list of exercises, but it gives you an idea of some of the easy activities we can do. Today's world is busy indeed, and we must use our spare moments. If you do only a few of the exercises daily, you're still better off than the person who doesn't exercise at all.

Also consider joining an exercise class. This can be an aerobics class, a conditioning class, karate lessons, or a group that walks together inside shopping malls. Peer pressure and the thought of others going through what you are somehow soothes the mind and makes exercise easier.

Whether you take a 30-minute walk or participate in a formal class of aerobics or karate, remember, diabetics need to exercise.

Chapter Fourteen

Brain Power and Positive Thinking

BY now you know I believe in a healthy, positive attitude. We should try to manage even the most negative sides of diabetes in a positive manner. Think about what happens when we deal with diabetes in a negative manner. We end up with a greater problem. Not only does the negative side of diabetes affect us, but the negative mind-set makes it worse.

I sincerely believe the old computer saying, "Garbage in, garbage out," applies to us, too. If you program for a negative result, most likely you'll get a negative result. On the other hand, if you program for a positive result, you'll be better able to handle whatever obstacle may occur, even it you don't fully reach your goal. Everything in life, including diabetes management, responds best to this positive mental attitude.

A French physician, Emile Cóué, came to America around 1920. He saw many sick people, and for many he wrote the same prescription: "Every day in every way, I am getting better, better, and better." He recommended that his patients repeat this prescription 20 times in the morning and 20 times before bed. This simple prescription achieved amazing results.

Positive thinking won't necessarily cause miracles. But remember, amazing events happen every day. Some say the insulin we use is a miracle. Yes, there are problems in living with diabetes, but who would prefer the alternative? Even diabetics who have lost eyes, kidneys, or legs will tell you they're better off than those who die because of poor diabetes management.

Brain Power

Albert Einstein, my hero since I was a child, said we only use 5 to 8 percent of our brain. Imagine what we could do if we double or triple the amount of brain we use? I've always wondered how the brain of a genius works. My brother Sam, who is four years younger than I am, is a natural genius. He was reading before the age of two. He could do math problems and write complex sentences when he was only three, and he was measured to have a genius I.Q.—over 168—at age six.

Sam finds better ways to do things and can do them in a special manner. When he asks me a question about medicine or diabetes, it's usually one I've never thought about. Sam is a special case. But, I do feel there is potential genius in each of us. The problem is we don't know how to use more of our brain.

The power of the mind is awesome, yet it remains untapped by many who are unaware of its positive energy. It's been found that those who preprogram themselves to die most certainly die. This doesn't mean those with the positive mind-set do not also die, but perhaps their quality of life is improved, even though it's their time to pass away. I believe this new area of medicine, where the mind is used to "cure" sickness, may someday be the new age of enlightened medicine.

Many scientists think the right brain is key to unleashing more brain power. The right brain is the intuitive side; the left brain is used more to accomplish our everyday tasks. Sensitive instruments have studied the role of brain frequencies. The brain is similar to a radio transmitter, operating on specific frequencies and voltages. At first, our brains function at the alpha brain wave frequency, a relatively mid-range frequency of about 7 to 14 cycles or hertz. As we move through adolescence and into adulthood, our brains run more in the beta range of frequencies, about 14 to 21 hertz and above.

Alpha Range

Researchers say the alpha range is the most beneficial brain wave. Beta brain wave functioning is adequate for everyday living, but for real problem solving capabilities, the alpha brain wave frequency is far superior. It is the frequency range where more of the genius qualities are derived.

Some say we can enter into an alpha state and instruct our brain to help heal our bodies, prepare for a test, or meet any of life's problems. A friend of mine taught me to use the right brain and alpha brain wave frequencies.

At the time, my diabetes had taken a turn for the worse, caused in part by the breakup of a close relationship. I was depressed and had a negative outlook. A routine blood chemistry, taken before I began working with my friend, showed my blood glucose levels were out of control. My cholesterol and blood fat levels were high. And my kidneys were in poor shape. What did I have to lose by trying something?

I began using the techniques of positive mind healing and right brain alpha states. Three months later, I had another blood chemistry. This time results were better than they'd been in years. My kidneys and blood glucose levels were excellent. My cholesterol had fallen below 200 mg/dl, and my blood fats were below 100 mg/dl. Everything looked so good that my doctor couldn't believe he was seeing the test results of a long-term, totally blind, diabetic patient.

Was this because of my right brain healing techniques? I can't say for sure. We still don't understand so many facets of the mind. However, the test results showed a great improvement over the previous ones and I was extremely happy.

Many books cover positive thinking techniques. Open your mind and study the various methods. I suggest reading the works of a pioneer in this field of study—Jose Silva. He created the Silva method of self-mind control over 25 years ago. He teaches that the right brain affects not only the physical self but also the mental and spiritual self.

Meditation

I also use total relaxation and meditation every day to create a complete sense of peace and tranquility. During these times I see myself in perfect health. Instead of envisioning diabetes leading to complications, I see myself repairing any damage in my body. Is this only wishful thinking? Remember, even with their high technology, scientists understand very little about the brain. And think about it: Are we too jaded and negative to believe that a miracle can happen to us?

A dear friend of mine, Betty Taylor, has written a special relaxation-meditation for me. I suggest you tape-record the meditation. Find a comfortable place, such as an easy chair, a reclining position on the floor, or lying on your bed. Play the tape recording and use a good pair of headphones so you can concentrate on the words and totally relax. The important goal is total relaxation. Concentrate on these words:

Close your eyes and take a deep relaxing breath. As you continue to breathe in and out, feel yourself relaxing, just relaxing, and going deeply within. Take another deep relaxing breath and be aware of the soft silence as your body begins to relax, one part at a time. Take another deep relaxing breath and exhale slowly. Feel your body relaxing from your head down to your toes. As you begin to relax more and more, and as you go deeper and deeper, you will feel a sense of drifting. Feel yourself floating and relaxing more and more with each breath that you take.

Imagine you are going to your favorite place of relaxation. Here you can be alone to renew and refresh yourself. You will be able to touch back into your deeper spiritual self. You will be able to feel a wonderful, perfect sense of well-being. Breathe gently in and out, and just drift with the sounds of your favorite place. This favorite place can be a spontaneously created place, or it can be a place from memory. It's only important that it be a secluded place; one where you can have the feeling of being away from the usual encroachments and stresses of life. As you go deeper and deeper into relaxation, you will want this special place to begin to appear clearly in your mind.

At this special place, it's always early in the morning, early dawn. This dawn represents the beginning of time and the beginning of you. You are now becoming part of this beginning of time. Begin to feel unburdened of worries, illness, and all the concerns and conflicts of life. Just release yourself from all the responsibilities you carry. Take a deep relaxing breath and exhale slowly. Let the rhythm of your breathing help you to go deeper and become more relaxed. Feel and sense the wonderful air of your favorite place. Feel a gentle breeze caress your hair and face. Take in another clean, refreshing breath and exhale slowly. Sense the sights, smells, and sounds of your special place. The more color and force you create in your imagination, the more of your mind you'll open for healing. This is your inner voyage, so make it as perfect as you want it to be.

Open your mind to the miracle of being alive. Fully appreciate the gift of life, no matter what the circumstances of your life may be. Feel contentment with yourself and appreciate the gift of being you. While your body continues to relax one part at a time, focus your attention in front of you and slightly raise your eyes to just above your horizontal plane of vision. Here you will find your mental screen.

On your mental screen, project an image of yourself. Concentrate on the muscles of your body. Picture the muscles of your body as being soft and loose, like rubber bands. Repeat mentally to yourself, "I ask my muscles to relax completely. All unnecessary tension and stress will leave my muscles, now." Picture all the blood vessels, arteries, capillaries, and smaller veins throughout your body. Sense the flow of blood through your body, feel the warmth of circulation, and repeat mentally to yourself, "I ask that my circulatory system carry all impurities out of my body and bring new life and vitality to all the cells in my body. My circulatory system is in complete harmony with all other systems of my body."

On your mental screen, imagine your respiratory system. Form a clear picture of your lungs. Watch the movements as your lungs expand to take in air and energy, and now, as your lungs contract, expel impurities from your body. Repeat mentally to yourself, "I ask that my respiratory system take in oxygen and use it efficiently. My respiratory system now carries cleansing oxygen into every area of my body. It's in harmony with all other systems of my body as it carries impurities away from all the cells of my body and outside of my system."

On your mental screen, form a picture of your digestive system. Imagine your stomach, pancreas, large intestine, small intestine, and colon. Repeat mentally to yourself, "I ask that my digestive system be in complete harmony within itself, with normal insulin-producing, healthy cells. My body now obtains the maximum good from all the food introduced into my body and rapidly expels the remainder out of my body as waste."

Form a mental picture of your kidneys. Visualize them working in harmony with all other parts of your body to eliminate waste. Repeat mentally to yourself, "I ask all impurities and excess fluids to pass quickly from my body."

Relax, take a deep breath, and go deeper. Visualize your heart on your mental screen. Add motion to this picture of your heart and hear it beating. Repeat mentally to yourself, "I ask that my heart be in perfect harmony within itself. My heart is now working at a top level of efficiency, neither overworking nor underworking. My heart is in complete harmony with all other systems of my body, causing all other systems of my body to work in a healthy manner."

On your mental screen, create an image of your skeletal system. Picture all the bones and joints in your body. Repeat mentally to yourself, "I ask all the bones and joints of my body to work with complete harmony within themselves. I ask all the unnecessary calcium deposits in my bones and joints, and elsewhere in my skeletal system, be dissolved and carried away from me. My joints now work at the utmost level of efficiency. The skeleton of my body is in perfect harmony with all other systems of my body."

Imagine yourself on your mental screen: the way you would look, reflecting perfect health, beauty, and weight. Enjoy this perfect picture of yourself. Every time you think of your health and appearance, you'll recall this image. Make this perfect image of yourself a blueprint for the way you wish to look and feel. This is your goal. This image is now you.

Repeat mentally these affirmations daily:

- All the systems of my body and mind are in complete harmony with themselves and each other.
- My higher self will maintain this balance by directing all the cells of my body that are created every day to restore and replace any cell that is diseased or injured with healthy cells. Through this process, my body will be kept in a state of perfect health where illness and injury are unable to exist.
- I'm a healthy, perfect human being in body, mind, and spirit.
- I'm in harmony with myself and the world I live in.
- Through my awareness and the power of my positive and energized mind, I am and shall continue to be a perfect, healthy human being.
- Every day, in every way, I am better, and better, and better.

The time is approaching for you to end this mental exercise. You may return to this place any time you wish just by closing your eyes and taking deep relaxing breaths. Better successes will follow when you repeat this mental exercise. Remember, it is you who is most important. As you come back to everyday awareness, be assured that you will be in your normal alert state, ready to attend to your daily duties with greater health, efficiency, and satisfaction. Be assured that you will feel stronger, healthier, happier, and more in harmony with yourself and the world you live in than before. Open your eyes.

Chapter Fifteen

On a Daily Basis

THIS conversation is meant to capture the moments after a young doctor has graduated from medical school. But the same words apply to a person with diabetes.

"Doctor, I trust your studies will help you give quality care to your patient," the wiser, experienced physician said with concern.

"Yes, sir, my training will assist me. But I lack experience with critical care situations. I think I'm plain afraid," the young doctor replied.

"Trust in your ability. You have studied and learned well. The only way to get experience is to get experience. Listen to the patient carefully and follow the rules of good practice. At all times, do what's best for the patient. And remember, medicine is a healing art, not an exact science. There is simply too much information for one person to know, but strive to understand the best techniques and latest theories, never forgetting the work carried out years ago," the old doctor lectured.

"I understand," the young doctor replied. "Do you have any more advice?"

"Know thyself. Treat thyself. Heal thyself. Look to the future and keep your eye on the now. I'll be here to help you when you need it. Good luck," the old doctor said with emotion. He knew his young colleague would be facing heights and depths in his new career.

Starting from the fright of diagnosis and the realization you must take insulin for the rest of your life to facing possible complications, managing your diabetes may be difficult. But progress is made when you decide you will not be defeated by this disease. Your determination to do the utmost, even in times of fear, will show your true character.

Diabetes is a full-time challenge. You can't take a break from it, so your strength must be high for the long haul. Yes, daily care can be challenging. That is why your doctor and the rest of the health care team are vital for good diabetes control. Try to stick to your management program and to think positively. Believe me, life is more difficult when you take a defeatist attitude. You are not a member of an exclusive club. Many people with diabetes are willing to discuss their management and coping techniques. Remain open to change. Allow yourself to make mistakes, but learn from them and try not to repeat them.

You may want to consider a career in science or medicine; you definitely have a vested interest. Creative thinking is critical for new theories and techniques in diabetes management.

I pray this book will help you meet the challenge of diabetes. Although you have read many of my thoughts, theories, and speculations concerning diabetes, these opinions are mine, based on more than 30 years of managing a rather severe case of Type 1 diabetes. This book is not a definitive thesis on diabetes. It is an introduction to the many challenges it can present. I hope you will benefit from my experiences, and from the challenge I place in your hands.

Reading List

The Diabetic Male's Essential Guide to Living Well by Joseph Juliano. Henry Holt & Company, 1998.

Diabetes: A Guide to Living Well, 3rd Edition by Gary Arsham and Ernest Lowe. Chronimed Publishing, 1997.

Diabetes: Questions You Have, Answers You Need by Paula Brisco. Peoples Medical Association Publishing, 1993.

Diabetes 101: A Pure and Simple Guide for People Who Use Insulin by Betty P. Brackenridge and Richard O. Dolinar. Chronimed Publishing, 1998.

Diabetes: Your Complete Exercise Guide by Neil F. Gordon. Human Kinetics Press, 1993.

Diabetes: A Practical New Guide to Healthy Living by James W. Anderson. Warner Books, 1991.

Weight Management for Type II Diabetes by Jackie Labat and Annette Maggi. Chronimed Publishing, 1997.

The Healing Journey by O. Carl Simonton and Reed M. Hanson. Bantam Books, 1992.

The Diabetic's Total Health Book, 3rd Edition by June Biermann and Barbara Toohey. JP Tarcher Publishing, 1992.

A Diabetic Doctor Looks at Diabetes: His and Yours by Peter Lodewick. RMI Corporation, 1988.

The Healing Brain: Breakthrough Discoveries about How the Brain Keeps Us Healthy by Robert Ornstein and David Sobel. Simon and Schuster, 1987.

Brain Power: A Neurosurgeon's Complete Program to Maintain and Enhance Brain Fitness throughout Your Life by Vernon Mark and Jeffery Piedmark. Houghton Mifflin, 1989.

Diabetes, Visual Impairment and Group Support: A Guide Book by Judith Caditz. Center for the Partially Sighted, 1989.

Super Potency by Dudley Danov. Time Warner, 1993.

Cooking and Nutrition

The Diabetic's Innovative Cookbook by Joseph Juliano and Dianne Young. Henry Holt, 1994.

Low Fat Living for Real People by Linda Levy and Francine Grabowski. Lake Isle Press, 1994.

Diabetic Low-Fat & No-Fat Meals in Minutes by M.J. Smith. Chronimed Publishing, 1996.

The Carbohydrate Counting Cookbook by Tami Ross and Patti Geil. Chronimed Publishing, 1998.

Eat More, Weigh Less by Dean Ornish. HarperCollins, 1993.

Family Cookbooks—4 Volumes from the American Diabetes Association and The American Dietetic Association.

Selected Magazines and Newspapers

The Voice of the Diabetic
Ed Bryant, editor
811 Cherry Street, Suite 309
Columbia, MO 65201

Diabetes Forecast
The American Diabetes Association, Inc.
Membership Services Division
P.O. Box 61054-0363
Mt. Morris, IL 61054

Diabetes Interview
3715 Balboa Street
San Francisco, CA 94121

Index

Also from Chronimed Publishing

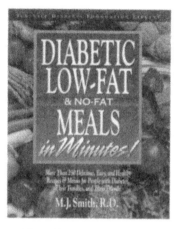

Diabetic Low-Fat & No-Fat Meals in Minutes
More than 250 Delicious, Easy, and Healthy Recipes & Menus for People with Diabetes, Their Families, and Their Friends

M.J. Smith, R.D.

From bestselling cookbook author M.J. Smith and the Juvenile Diabetes Foundation—the world's leading health agency funding diabetes research—comes this deluxe, hardcover cookbook with 16 pages of full color photographs and over 250 recipes for tantalizing all-American favorites from breakfasts to desserts. Most recipes take under 30 minutes to prepare, and the ingredients can be found in virtually any grocery store. The book also includes diabetic menus for 60 days. Plus, each recipe features a complete nutrition analysis, including diabetic exchanges.

1-56561-084-9 • $24.95

Available at your favorite bookstore.

Also from Chronimed Publishing

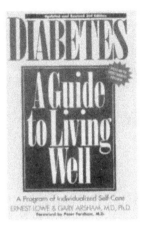

Diabetes: A Guide to Living Well
Third Edition
Ernest Lowe and Gary Arsham, M.D., PhD.

Diabetes A Guide to Living Well incorporates new information, emphasizing the current focus on preventive measure to avoid common major complications, such as insulin reaction and hyperglycemia. This important information is supported by the results of the Diabetes Control and Complications Trial completed in 1993, proving that an intensive regimen of frequent blood glucose tests along with appropriate diet and insulin adjustments does in fact reduce the risks of long-term complications.

1-56561-112-8 • $14.95

Available at your favorite bookstore.

Check out our website for other health-related titles
CHRONIMED PUBLISHING
www.chronimed.com

Also from Chronimed Publishing

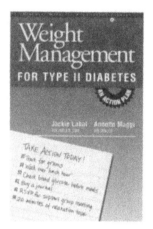

Weight Management for Type II Diabetes
An Action Plan

Jackie Labat, M.S., R.D., C.D.E. and Annette Maggi, M.S., R.D.

This is the first resource combining nutrition and exercise information specifically for people with Type II diabetes, including: setting reasonable exercise goals; keeping pace with an exercise regimen; learning to deal with lapses; developing lifestyle habits that last; managing stress; teaming up with others for support; and handling special occasions.

1-56561-114-4 • $12.95

Available at your favorite bookstore.

Also from Chronimed Publishing

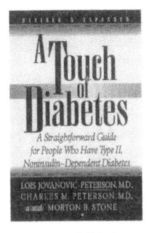

A Touch of Diabetes
A Straightforward Guide for People who have
Type II, Noninsulin-Dependent Diabetes
Revised and Expanded

Lois Jovanovic-Peterson, M.D.,
Charles M. Peterson, M.D.,
and Morton B. Stone

Everything people with newly-diagnosed noninsulin-dependent diabetes need to know, from curbing potential complications to counting calories, is in this authoritative and easy-to-understand guide.

1-56561-079-2 • $10.95

Available at your favorite bookstore.

Also from Chronimed Publishing

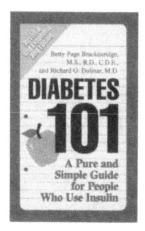

Diabetes 101
A Pure and Simple Guide for People Who Use Insulin

Betty Page Brackenridge, M.S., R.D., C.D.E.,
and Richard O. Dolinar, M.D.

This clear and breezy guide, written by two of the most acclaimed experts in diabetes care and education, uses real-life examples in an engaging story format that's fun to read. *Diabetes 101* answers the questions that every person with diabetes has.

Available at your favorite bookstore.

Check out our website for other health-related titles
CHRONIMED PUBLISHING
www.chronimed.com